NO WORRIES

Towards glow &
effective worrying

Bryn Jones

A Snowdragon Book

First published 2018 by H B Jones, Welshpool, Wales

ISBN: 978-1721969678

This book is no substitute for a health practitioner. If worry is making you ill, go and see a health practitioner.

Cover designed and book typeset in Minion Pro & Helvetica Neue by Edda Salander-Jones

Printed by CreateSpace

Dedicated, with no more but my

love,

to my daughter Edda.

This is to acknowledge my heartfelt

gratitude

to those countless patients and clients over the years who have helped to make my working life a glorious adventure.

Contents

war

1 THE BEGINNING

**How a little boy learnt to stop feeling
and learn about war.**

War is a dangerous adventure. That is what the little boy
thought as he woke up in a huge room among 103 sick
and dying grown up men.

The lump on his neck, the size of an egg, was hurting a
bit, the men's coughing made a horrible sound and he was
afraid. Afraid of what? He did not know, except that the
doctor had told him that he would here for some time and
that he would get better and the lump would go away but
only if he behaved himself. It was wartime, 1944 in a TB
Sanatorium in the moorlands of Wales, Great Britain. The
nurses not only had to look after the grown up tubercular
men and him but were also responsible for nursing dozens
of wounded soldiers waiting to return home to Canada
after losing arms or legs in the War.

The little boy was expected to be brave, very brave and not
cry and not make a fuss about anything. All because of the
War.

Now, the little boy did not really understand what War was, he was just 5 years old and some months ago his father took him to the top of a hill near his home in the evening and showed him a huge fire in the distance and said, "That is Liverpool burning because of the bombs dropped by the Germans". It looked very spectacular, just like the bonfire on Guy Fawkes Day but this was during the month of April not the 5th of November.

But he was still afraid. It was early morning, very dark, some of the men were snoring, others coughing their guts out (or so it sounded) and he was very much alone and missed his mother, his father and his home. He was also very worried that he would not be able to stop crying in front of the nurses.

Sound is a very special sense. You can close your eyes and your mouth but you cannot close your ears. Sound comes in to you whether you want it or not. Of course, some sounds are very pleasant and we want more of them, like good music. Other sounds are not pleasant, they disturb our inner sense of harmony, they grate, they make us feel uncomfortable. Just like the tubercular, racking, coughing sounds coming from these adult men all around the little boy. These coughing sounds entered into every single cell of this young body and made him feel that his body was breaking apart. It was very frightening.

If all goes well, adults are, for little children, all-powerful and all-knowing, but if something goes wrong it can be very disconcerting. So being all alone in this huge open ward full of adult men, all of whom were ill and some of whom were dying, was very disorienting and frightening for the little boy. Even more so because there was no escape. No getting away from the sounds, the smells, the presence of illness and death.

Quite horrible, really.

But then it was winter and all of a sudden everything outside was covered in snow. The large ward with the 103 sick and dying men and the one little boy had big glass sliding doors leading out to a big terrace. One day, the sun came out and the little boy, still in his bed, was wheeled out on to the terrace with men in their beds and each was given a bucket filled with snow and they had a snowball fight on the terrace. All the beds and all the people were covered in snow and everyone laughed and had a good time, including the little boy who could not remember ever having had such fun in the snow.

Discipline was something that Nurse R. was very good at. She also did her best to ensure that the little boy learnt to be disciplined by explaining to him the ground rules according to which he had to behave.

If he played the game correctly he would become healthy and could later go home and play and go to school like all the other children. The rules were:

Do not cry.

Only speak when you are spoken to.

Be quiet.

Do as you are told by the doctors and nurses.

Only then can you go home.

Nurse R. explained that in the building next door there were lots of soldiers from Canada who had been wounded during the War and had lost a leg or an arm and were at the Sanatorium to convalesce before going home at the end of the War. The little boy should realise that these soldiers almost gave their lives to protect the little boy and his parents from the evil Germans who had been bombing the British towns and people in order to force them to surrender. But they were not going to surrender. Mr Churchill had made that clear to the whole world. And so the little boy had to do his duty, play by the rules and behave. Then he would slowly get healthy and be able to go home and live in peace at the end of the War.

The real boss of the Sanatorium was Matron. The doctors came and went, some of them to other hospitals, some of them went to War but Matron stayed here. She was a very handsome and strict person and exuded authority and power. Kindness was not part of her personal vocabulary.

One day she summoned the little boy to her office and informed him that the enemy had sunk the ship that was bringing modern new machines from America, three of which were destined for the Sanatorium. They were artificial light machines specifically designed to heal people like him, suffering from Tuberculosis. Sadly, the evil Germans had thwarted those plans. Now all would have to wait for the next shipment and that could take many months because of the War. The little boy would have to be very patient but Matron had some good news for him: one of the wounded soldiers was a trained teacher and would help the little boy by teaching him to read and write. "But Matron, I can read and write" said the little boy. "Yes, but you can only read and write Welsh …", said Matron "and the new teacher will teach you English."

Thus a whole new world opened up for the little boy because he was then slowly able to get to know the wounded soldiers and heard all sorts of stories from them about the War and the Continent.

Then two other little boys arrived at the Sanatorium and the soldiers came to visit and brought oranges, chewing gum and 'Crunchy' bars with them. The boys loved the soldiers and heard from them that there was another building nearby with girl and women patients.

Death is a strange thing for a five year old. One day the little boy was visiting the building where his soldier-teacher was and on the way he had to go to the loo. So he looked for the nearest toilet and went in. There, on the floor, lying very still was a little girl just about his age. He had never seen her before. In fact he had, at this point in time, not seen any of the girls that were said to be in the hospital. But there was no doubt about the fact that lying in front of him on the floor was a little girl and she was not moving at all. He went to her and shook her a bit but she did not respond so he just went back to the corridor to look for a nurse. He found one and told her what happened and showed her the toilet. The nurse just took one look at the little girl and gave the little boy to another nurse who took him back to his own bed.

Later on one of the men patients said that the little boy was very brave and that it was such a shame that the little girl was dead. Well, the little boy was curious and a bit afraid when he heard that because, up to now, he had only heard about soldiers dying in the War. Since he had been told to not disturb anyone he was even afraid to ask anyone how it happened that a little girl could die. She just looked asleep but she did not move. And now he knew that she was not asleep. She was just dead. He started to be a little bit afraid but not really; he was just desperate to talk to someone.

So he went for a walk to his favourite place, under the trees near the goldfish pond. Once there he thought it might be a good idea to talk to the goldfish. Of course he knew that they could not talk back to him but they did seem very calm and content and they might well be prepared to listen to him. So he started to talk to them about what happened with him and the little girl and after a while he began to feel better, said good-bye to the goldfish and went back to his bed and his toys.

That was the beginning of a long and satisfying friendship with the goldfish in the fishpond and this was where he went when he wanted to share his secret thoughts without being told to behave himself and be quiet.

One day one of the doctors came to the little boy and told him that he would be getting an operation on his neck and that he would go to sleep and when he woke up the big lump on his neck, by now it was as big as an egg, would be gone. Then he would be treated with the new lamps from America and slowly he would be a healthy little boy again.

Sounded good but strange, why did he have to go to a theatre of all places? What kind of theatre is an Operating Theatre? All very weird. Anyway the next morning he was taken to the theatre and laid on a couch under a very big and very bright lamp; a piece of gauze cloth was put over his nose and mouth and drops of some liquid came down. At the same time the lamp started to move and rotate and he felt drawn up into it and started turning in circles inside the lamp and then felt as if he was falling upwards into the lamp and then, just blackness, peace and nothing.

Sometime later he woke up in his own bed with a bandage around his neck and Nurse K. smiling at him and asking if he was OK. Then she went off and came back with a big ice cream for the little boy. He was very happy, it was his first ice cream since coming to the hospital. Then the doctor came and said that he was a very good patient and how did he like the going to sleep. They both laughed as he described his falling up rather than falling down and then they left him alone with his ice cream.

Even though it was Spring it was still quite cold but the ice cream tasted very delicious and the little boy loved Nurse K. who had brought him the ice cream. She was always coming by to ask how he was and to admire the things he was making with cardboard, scissors and glue.

The first few days after the operation were not pleasant. The little boy's neck was quite sore, particularly when he moved his head but he was very happy when he had visitors. Every day Nurse K. stopped by and then every afternoon one or two of the wounded soldiers came by bringing gifts of sweets or fruit and sometimes comics. The visitors also gave him the opportunity to show off his farm. Yes he had built a wall, a farmhouse and a barn and stuck them all to a piece of plywood. The problem of farm animals was solved by catching 'daddy longlegs' insects and fastening a little ball of Plasticine to their legs so that they could not get over the farm wall. Sometimes dead flies had to take the place of pigs on the farm. Most of the visitors seemed to be fascinated by the little boy's farm particularly when they heard that he let the daddy longlegs out every evening by removing the Plasticine. He did not tell them that sometimes he had to remove a leg because the Plasticine got stuck!

The next day he started all over again, collecting live daddy longlegs insects and dead flies.

The little boy liked Nurse K. very much. She was always kind to him, she always came by when she was near, just to say 'hello' and she was very tender and careful when she had to do something to him, whether washing him or changing one of the dressings on his wound after an operation.

In other words, the little boy loved Nurse K. That was not really surprising because she was the only person around who gave him any kind of physically expressed loving care and attention. Otherwise he was often starving from lack of love. The sick men patients and the two older boys were much too concerned with their own illnesses to be able to spend time with the lonely little boy.

The teacher seemed to enjoy the few hours he spent each week with his young pupil but was otherwise very busy getting fit and healthy again as well as having to work a lot with helping the other soldiers, particularly the ones who were not yet able to move around.

The little boy was now recovering well from his first operation and the new healing lamps had finally arrived from America, so he was slowly getting better and could in fact move around quite freely around the Sanatorium and the grounds. Now that he could read English he was always on the lookout for things to read, books, magazines, newspapers, comics, it did not matter what it was as long as he had something to read. When the weather was nice he went down to the fishpond, made himself comfortable, and read and spoke to his friends the goldfish about what he had learnt.

War seemed very far away for the little boy. He remembered being told how Father woke up one morning in his hotel in London and a house next door was a pile of debris, a bomb had fallen on it during the night. He was also told about the bombs that destroyed Coventry, a large town near which his Aunt and Uncle lived. War for him seemed to be all about bombs and fire and large towns.

When he came to the Sanatorium, things changed. There was no cinema, no TV, no radio, no newspapers (at least not for little boys), just a lot of soldiers who were hurt during and because of the War. Then he slowly began to read the comics, mostly American comics, and saw pictures, horrible pictures, of Nazis and Japanese villains doing terrible things to the Allied soldiers when they caught them and made them prisoners. These were the stories of the ones who got away. Then there were the stories from the wounded soldiers that he saw every day. They told him about falling out of burning aeroplanes, of jumping out of shot-up tanks, of being hit by a bullet or a shell in a trench. Then one day he was shown a map of Europe and how the soldiers had to be flown or transported on ships before they could start to fight. It all seemed very complicated, but then he was told that it really was very simple. On the one side was Hitler, he was very, very bad and on the other side, our side, was Mr Churchill. Now he was a very good leader, he made sure that Hitler lost the war and tomorrow they were all going to have a big party to celebrate Victory in Europe. The little boy was asked to help by gathering as much dead wood that he could find for the bonfire.

The next day all was ready. A huge effigy of Hitler had been made and put on top of a huge bonfire. In the evening the bonfire was lit and everyone cheered as Hitler was burnt.

The little boy was very happy. Victory seemed to be a good thing because everyone was smiling and happy. He was also happy because Father and Mother were coming to visit the next day and he had lots to tell them.

His parents' visit was the highlight of the little boy's week. He had been told from the very beginning that because of the War and the Rationing, his parents could only come to visit him once a week on Sunday afternoon. He missed them a lot but he was also very proud that he had learnt to be very brave and not complain and certainly not cry, even though it was sometimes very hard not to.

The visit was restricted to three hours and sometimes other relatives or friends came with Mummy and Daddy. Often they played some new game that had been brought, or they looked at some of the new books that arrived. If the weather was friendly they all went for a little walk in the grounds but the little boy tried to make sure that they did not go near the fishpond, he wanted to keep the goldfish his own little secret. Often the time went very quickly and then the little boy had to fight very hard not to cry when it was time for them to leave. The next day one of the soldiers was sure to come by and give him an orange or some chewing gum, which he then promptly exchanged for a Crunchy bar, his absolute favourite piece of chocolate.

Sometimes the soldiers spoke about the War and the Nazis and how evil they were and how it would be a very good thing for Europe when the War was finally over and the British and the Americans could help build up Europe again.

But the little boy was more concerned about getting healthy and spent every second day under the health lamps until one day Matron told him that he was now well enough to go home. It was almost 12 months since he first came to the Sanatorium, the War was over, he was a year older and healthy and he could not wait to go home.

Then the big day came and the car arrived with his Mummy and Daddy to carry the little boy home. What an adventure. Yes indeed, after a little while the whole stay in the Sanatorium began to feel like a huge adventure, everyone was interested in what happened and the grown ups were amazed to hear the little boy speaking such good English.

On the other hand the children soon found out that he was not very strong and that he was quite sickly so that he could not play lots of the rough games that the boys loved. And so three years went by with the little boy spending lots of time constructing things with his Meccano set and playing with his toy railway.

Then one horrible day he felt a lump in his tummy which was followed by months and months of going to a doctor who looked like a Nazi and who stuck metal things into his bottom that hurt a lot but, because he was well trained, he did not cry and did not tell anyone how much it hurt.

After six months he was told that he was to have another operation, but since the two operations in the Sanatorium did not hurt very much he was not at all worried.

That was a bad mistake.

The operation went well and did not hurt because of course he was anaesthetised, but afterwards it was horrendous. One day he looked at the wound as Nurse was changing the dressing and got a shock, it was half open with blood clots, it was huge, going on for about 10 cm. and had six big metal things holding it together. Then the next week he was told that they were going to remove the metal clips, that it was going to hurt, that he would not get any anaesthetic because he was a brave patient and that they were going to do it over a few days and not all at once.

There followed a week of that was perceived by the ten year old boy as "torture". However, it was 'for his own good", 'children don't feel pain as much as adults and forget very quickly' and it was just after the war.

As you have probably guessed by now, that little boy is the author of this book.

I decided to write about my early experiences because I have, during hundreds of hours of personal and training analysis, both individual and group, and more than 30 years of practising psychotherapy, learnt that such experiences, once they have been allowed to become conscious and 'worked through' in a safe and secure setting, can form a very stable and secure foundation and help develop valuable empathic feelings towards the sufferings of other human beings on this earth.

big
bang

2 PERSPECTIVES

About the importance of viewpoints.

Health has been uppermost in my unconscious mind since I was 18 months old and had to spend three weeks in an isolation ward in a local hospital because of an unknown fever sickness; and in my conscious mind since the age of six, when I had to go to a TB Sanatorium in the Welsh Moorlands, during World War Two, to be treated for an illness called 'Bovine TB', a form of tuberculosis transmitted through milk.

I hope that this book will appeal to, and be useful for, those increasing numbers of people who are open to looking at life from a different perspective.

People who don't longer think in terms of the bigger the better, people who are really concerned about what is happening to the earth, to the oceans, to our air, to our water and who are very concerned about the inheritance they are going to leave behind. This book is for those people with those types of concerns because they are particularly prone to converting their concern into worry, sometimes to the point of harming themselves and their personal environment through excessive worrying and through relationship behaviour based on repressed anxiety.

Adolf Guggenbuhl-Craig was a Swiss Psychoanalyst whom I met whilst studying Jungian Analysis in Zurich in the late 1970s. I found him, in contrast to many of the other analysts, a very warm person. He had recently had a major heart attack and one of his close friends told me that he was a different human being afterwards!

So, as you can imagine, I was quite intrigued by this and it inspired me to look closer. Not only at the difficulties I had always had with breathing deeply and the question of connections between breathing more deeply and being a warm and open person, but also at the powerful effect a long fast, mainly on fruit juices, that I had just undergone, was having on my capacity to breath more deeply.

It was more than 25 years later, after an open-heart surgical operation leading to a new, artificial aorta valve that it was found that I was born with a defect valve and that the valve opening had slowly 'clogged up'. However, all arteries, heart muscles etc. were in very good condition!

It took many months before I was able to work again, I became quite depressed and decided to undergo another major psychoanalysis.

Strange though it may sound, the stay in the heart hospital was very healing for me and helped me work through the various hospitalisation traumas, starting with the ones noted above at the ages of 18 months and six years as well as the major trauma after a stomach operation for Crohn's Disease at the age of 10 where they removed eight steel clips from the wound without any anaesthetic.

During the analysis I was often reminded about Guggen-buhl-Craig and his ability, many years ago, to transform his own trauma into an act of loving kindness. Sadly, he died in 2008, just a couple of years before I began writing these lines.

One of the issues was came up during analysis was the stomach surgery. Crohn's Disease is particularly unpleas-ant because it attacks the area where the small gut joins the colon. It often leads to pain as well as loss of bowel control. Not at all a good thing for a 10 year old boy. Nowadays it is treated with medication and psychothera-py. In the UK in the late 1940s there was only one option; surgical removal of part of the inflamed gut, with around 50:50 chance of survival into middle age.

The operation itself was painless; I was, after all, under anaesthesia, but the aftermath was horrific. The wound, about 10 cm. long was closed with eight steel clips, each clip being a much larger version of the wire staples used to hold paper together. Every movement was painful. Then came the day to remove the clips. No anaesthetic. It was decided to spread the action over a few days. The nurses were sympathetic but very decisive. The doctor was brusque and not very sympathetic. The decision was made to remove between one and three clips each time with two days break in between. Just try to imagine how it feels to have even a small wire staple removed from an unhealed wound. I only have a vague recollection of how my reaction but I do remember one young nurse saying that my crying with pain was too much for her and asked to be excused.

At the end of the week all the clips were out and there was just a dull aching pain where they had been. Within a month that pain also went away so that there was only the memory. But that was enough for me to promise myself that I would never ever again say anything that could possibly bring me into a hospital where they could do such horrible painful things.

I learnt over the years to hide all signs of pain and hurt. But unfortunately, quite unconsciously, I also learnt to hide, even from myself, all the emotional pains and hurts that play such an important role in healthy and intimate human relationships.

It took many years and lots of therapeutic help before I was able to openly show any signs of pain, whether physical or emotional.

At the age of 15 I taught myself self-hypnosis to control the pain that sometimes came unexpected. I was absolutely certain that come what may no one would be able to suspect that I was in pain and so there was no danger of my being forced again to go into hospital for surgery, no way was I going to give 'them' an excuse to open me up again!

At 18 years of age I left home to study, learnt about using alcohol and drugs as pain-killers, worked as a design engineer, got married (no children, and a friendly divorce), moved on to conceive, plan and manage trade fairs and ended up designing and building 'Gwynedd 69', a major trade/cultural event to celebrate the Investiture of Charles as Prince of Wales in Caernarfon, Wales in 1969.

Then came my own personal 'Big Bang'.

I discovered meditation, Vipassana Meditation. After discovering that giving up my career as a successful young, creative manager in the trade fair industry, living on a vegetarian diet, hardly any alcohol, no cigarettes and hardly any drugs were having a very positive effect on my health, I attended a series of lectures at the Buddhist Society in

London and took part in a 10 week course in meditation. After some months of practice, I had a particularly awesome experience, which I can only describe as 'being frozen in a moment of time in a ball of light'. Very strange, particularly for someone who had studied mechanical engineering!

Then came the wild years, earning money as a freelancer introducing humanistic psychology and encounter groups to London through the first Human Growth Centre in Europe, based on the model of the Esalen Institute in California. Training as a Naturopath, healing myself, learning to heal others, further training in group work, living for short periods in Deya, Majorca and Paris, France, visiting New York, and Big Sur, being friends with amazing people like Gerda Boyesen, John and Eva Pierrakos, Paul Lowe, Carolee Schneeman, John Lifton, Mitsou Naslednikov, later better known as Margot Anand, George King and John Drane. Then founding The Works in Fulham, London with Joanna Cock whom I later married and with whom we had a daughter Edda. Living in The Common House with up to about 14 other people and great house parties with people like John Robinson who declared God to be dead, the musicians Remy Kabaka and Steve Winwood, dancers like Xenia Hribar from Contemporary Dance Company. Michael Wynne-Williams coming up from Wales in between fighting for the fledgling Green consciousness. Commuting between London, Zurich, Switzerland and Frankfurt/Main, Germany to earn money and study Jungian Psychoanalysis, before finally settling down in Germany in 1981, building up a private psychotherapy practice, losing a lot of money on a crazy building project in the 'Westerwald', a loving divorce from Joanna, marriage again to Jana Marinova, a Bulgarian living in Germany since 1979. Charity work in Bulgaria, a major heart operation, closing down my practice office in

Frankfurt, living partly in Sofia, Bulgaria, partly in Wales, spending time in India and Bali, before deciding to, at last, write this book.

Time as a concept has always fascinated me since my prolonged stay, of about 12 months, in the TB Sanatorium on the Denbigh Moors at the end of World War II. As a six-year old you don't have much of a sense of time. After all, being promised that you will leave this place in a few months meant just the same as 'never'.

A big stone sitting peacefully on top of a mountain contains lots of potential energy. If at some period in time it starts to move, particularly if it starts to move downwards, the combination can be very powerful in terms of converting the potential into dynamic energy, as those unfortunate people find out if they happen to be in the path of an avalanche.

Potential is something that we all have in common. The potential to be; the potential to become; the potential to do.

In the last few years something quite amazing has been going on in mainstream science .... people are talking about the concept of instantaneous change, the immediate transformation of potential into reality and potential forms and images coming into being instantaneously with no time lag between chaos and order.

In my particular case it took about 25 years of calendar time between my stay in a small restricted space for a year at the sanatorium and the 'big bang' experience described above. It was only then that I even began to perceive of the vast amount of potential energy lurking inside of me.

Then around 12 and half years of calendar time to begin the process of healing, of in-corpo-ration ... the integration of my body into my being ... of learning to look at situations and processes consciously from another perspective. A fascinating and fantastic time.

Physics, particularly quantum physics has developed a great deal in the last 50 years. As far as I can understand, one new theory is that it is no longer a question of an electron being either wave or particle, they are both! I saw a demonstration recently whereby it started off with a chaotic, random pattern of particles that at some point transformed into a wave pattern. Not only that, the transformation occurred instantaneously. It reminded me of how an Asian butterfly thousand of miles away can, at the same time, influence a climatic process in the heart of Europe.

Not only that, but it seems to have something to do with the concept of an immanent form which, under particular circumstances, can change in an instant, with no time lag, from a potential form into a real form.

Just think how amazing it would be if you, yes, you personally, had, tucked away somewhere inside you, a secret, potential form of yourself that could just be waiting for the opportunity to change into a real form.

Small changes in a human person are usually associated, particularly in the areas of personality, consciousness, character etc. with happening over a particular stretch of time, whereas bodily changes particularly in the areas of sickness are widely accepted as being able to manifest instantaneously, e.g. a heart attack or a stroke. Interesting don't you think?

A quantum leap, at least in the everyday sense as opposed to the strictly scientific, usually refers to an instantaneous revolutionary change. Now in the realms of consciousness there are lots of examples of this type of change. For instance Archimedes, the ancient Greek scholar, shouted 'eureka' out loud as he was having a bath and, in one second, discovered the Archimedes Principle regarding an exact precise method of measuring the volume of irregularly shaped masses and thus solved a problem that had been a puzzle since the dawn of civilisation. He apparently was so excited that he ran through the streets naked to proclaim his discovery!

A lot of people have the experience of a sudden, intuitive flash that helps them solve a problem and the work of people like Erik Kandel a recipient of the Nobel Prize is devoted to exploring the interaction between conscious and unconscious memory processes that could be behind such instant learning examples.

Ancient Indian philosophies also spoke of the possibility of an instant transformation in consciousness.

What is in general still not clear is whether one can consciously learn how to prepare for such processes, whether through purely intellectual thought process, through deep psychological, analytical processes or through various forms of meditation. At one time or another, I have experimented with all three methods and hope to share with you in this book some of my insights into this question.

Emotional feeling is something special. It's different to a bodily feeling but at the same time it is closely linked to bodily feeling. For instance, a sudden noise can remind you, because of its particular sound quality, sometimes just below the level of normal consciousness, of an event that was associated with feelings of strong anxiety and fearfulness. It can then trigger off a quickening of the heart pulse rate before eventually manifesting itself as an emotional feeling of being anxious or even afraid. Only then do you notice the increased heart pulse and think of it as being a reaction to being afraid and not the other way round.

So the interaction between emotional and bodily feelings is often quite complex and has been the subject of a lot of interesting scientific and not so scientific theories.

For instance, one serious subject of scientific research is laughing. Dr William Fry has been researching the subject at Stanford University, USA and his findings have been used in Japan to start classes in learning how to laugh so that people can then learn to relax and eventually be more content and even happier in their lives.

Thus it is not always the case that we laugh because we are happy. Consider laughing in order to become happy, a kind of reverse engineering of the soul.

While the transformation of seeing something funny makes us laugh almost immediately, the process of transforming laughter, a basically bodily process, into an emotional feeling like happiness has to be learned and can take some time, but might well be worth trying, particularly if you have been brought up in a culture that did not encourage laughter. Germany in the 1980s was certainly not a welcoming place to laugh in. Laughter was not 'serious' and therefore not acceptable. Fortunately things have now changed in Germany. But in Japan there are special classes in learning how to laugh in order to be more relaxed.

Does the above remind you of 'positive thinking'? In the 1930s and in fact well up to the 1960s, books about 'positive thinking' were very popular. It all started of course with Dale Carnegie even though Victorian times were influenced by a Frenchman called Coue who propagated a mantra around the idea of how to get healthy by saying and believing in 'every day a little bit better'.

Dale Carnegie's ideas sound a bit dated from our point of view but his writings on the art of public speaking are still very sound. Society has changed enormously since the 1930s and we now know much more about the important role of emotional intelligence and particularly about how the abilities to look at, to express, to analyse and to judge the effectiveness of expressing our emotions in terms of relating to others.

Society is now different. Public and social issues are so different to how they were. Lateral structures are more effective than rigid hierarchical structures. Just look at the difference between Apple and General Motors. Daily life is not only more complex it also changes unbelievably fast compared to even 50 years ago.

Do you always get what you want? Beware! One of the dangers of getting what you want is that you might just get it. Which may be OK if you are prepared for it. However mostly it happens that people are not prepared for it. This is amusingly and instructively illustrated in some of the tales written by Wilhelm Hauff, a German writer in the 1890s.

There is one in particular that deals with a couple that are visited by a good fairy who grants them 3 wishes. They start arguing about which three wishes to present and in the middle of the argument the wife became exasperated and said "Gosh I just wish we had a big plate of sausages and could eat them in peace and quiet". All of a sudden, there it was, a big plate full of sausages on the table between them. Then the husband got angry and said, "You silly old goose, you're going to spoil it all with your big mouth, I really do wish that one of those sausages grows out of your nose!" Well, guess what, yes that also happened so that they had no choice but to use the very last of the three wishes to get rid of the sausage growing out of her nose.

You see, there is indeed a danger in getting too involved in dreaming about things that you wish for. It's always better to make plans for getting what you want rather than using a lot of energy in determining what you would do if you got it.

Some people seem to feel quite at home with a chaotic environment. Just have a look at your desk, work-bench, kitchen table or dressing table to determine whether you are one of them.

But very often what seems to an outsider to be chaotic is for the owner/user not at all, they have their own way of dealing with the bits and pieces. Sometimes they take more time, sometimes less but it is rare that they get thrown off course by the seemingly chaotic arrangement of their things.

Robert was a very successful but rather eccentric lawyer whose small desk was usually empty apart from the one case he was working on at that moment. However the whole floor of his office as well as most of the chairs and occasional tables were covered with stacks of files that nobody else was allowed to move. It looked like complete chaos but he had his own system and it worked for him, as I said, he was indeed successful at his work. In Robert's conscious mind there was very little chaos and a lot of clarity and he was able to process the sometimes enormous amount of seemingly unrelated facts to find the underlying pattern.

Then there are other people whose thoughts, ideas and worries are indeed very chaotic inside them and often give cause for conflict in terms of getting things done. They keep on getting sidetracked and end up a long way from the dream goal.

If you, dear reader, are one of them, try writing it down. That is, get it out of your mind and on to paper or PC or Mac or iPad or even a cell phone. Express your concerns and your ideas, your thoughts and your feelings, your dreams and your worries. You may well be a very creative person who just has to learn about construction.

To drop out was a very popular phrase in the 1960s. Often it was used to represent young people who had studied or worked and found little deep satisfaction in what they were doing and who were attracted to various alternative lifestyles that were beginning to be represented in the 'Western Media'.

In the United Kingdom these alternatives can be broadly classified by three words. The Beatles, Carnaby Street and Hippy. The first, 'Beatles', was of course the name of the music group of John Lennon, Paul MacCartney, Ringo Starr and George Harrison. But it also meant more than that, it also meant pop music, dancing in the streets, soft drugs, music festivals, pirate radio; the first careful coming together of classical and light music and much more. The second word 'Carnaby Street' was actually the name of a little shopping street in the West End of London but came to stand for a revolutionary change in the world of fashion and design as well as art. But the third 'Hippy' came to mean love and peace, a new form of spirituality as well as a love of nature. It meant Glastonbury, not just the festival, Buddhism, a strange, dream-like relationship between the Police and some of the 'drop outs', sometimes even worthy of the adjective 'magical'. But that's a long time ago now.

As a successful young manager with a proven track record in the world of international trade fairs it was very easy for me to decide to drop out. In those days it was very easy to reverse the decision and get back into the rat race. Not at all like 2014, where taking a long break often means it is almost impossible to get back.

Well, my own dropping out lead me all over the world, to study natural therapy in California, Slovenia and Ceylon, mediation in India and London and psycho analysis in Switzerland. From creative chaos to an established private psychotherapy practice in Germany.

Individual is a word that describes something or someone quite unique. For instance, contrary to a widely spread opinion, individual human beings are quite different from the instance of birth, except of course for the special case of twins. Apart from the possible different colour of their skin, individual human beings are also different by virtue of things like interests, capabilities and talents.

Then there are different nations of peoples. They also differ from each other, usually through cultural trends or characteristics.

My own particular cultural, national background is Welsh, specifically the Welsh speaking North West corner centred around Caernarfon and Snowdonia, the land of the mythical and of the real King Arthur and of Merlin. The land of the Druids, of poets and musicians, of the British Prime Minister David Lloyd George, the footballer Gareth Beal, the film stars Richard Burton, Catherine Zeta-Jones and Anthony Hopkins as well as the pop music groups Super Furry Animals and Manic Street Preachers The language is Cymraeg, one of the oldest living European languages, a Celtic language related to Gaelic and Breton with a colourful cultural history.

We were always a cultural minority. That sometimes gives us a deep empathy towards minorities. Sometimes also an antipathy.

Then of course there is something else, there is a global
movement that is best described by the word Tribes. It is
very much a product of this Age of Instant Communication. Sometimes short-lived, sometimes showing signs
of getting established for some time, it is a movement of
people, mostly young at heart, often young in age, but
always joined by a hard to define thread which constantly
takes on different forms, colours and tastes. Sometimes
the community is linked through Apple, iPhone and iPad
users, sometimes centred around climate change issues.
The interesting thing about it is that it often transcends
global, national boundaries and even though the original
language was English there are myriads of tribes using
other languages and dialects. However the one common
thread is Internet, the constantly growing world-wide-web
of data connections morphing into mobile phones, com-
puters, TVs, tablets and so on, whenever appropriate.

Please bear all that in mind when reading this book, it
is certainly not designed for the mainstream, not for the
Readers Digest type (huh! does it really still exist?). It is
designed for people who like to look around corners, who
are open to an experimental approach to life, an approach
based on experience and not on theoretical or dogmatic
principles.

I do hope you enjoy it and that even if there is nothing
new for you here, then let's hope that it will serve as a
timely reminder to really do something with or about the
knowledge and experience that you have. And please don't
forget that at a very early age you actually did learn, all
alone, to utter the first words, to take the first steps as well
as to shed the first tears without the help of a manual or a
coach.

Are friends important for you? You may well respond by
saying that is a rather stupid question because most people

treasure friends. But there again not everyone does. So let me ask another question. What is so special, so different, about friends? John MacMurray, a Scots Quaker philosopher once said that the most important characteristic about friendship is time. Yes, time; because that is really the one and only thing that you can justifiably demand from a friend, that they share their time with you. Money, sport, hobbies, respect, advice, even love, are not central to friendship, but time certainly is, particularly in an emergency.

We were referring above to friends with a small 'f'. What about Friends, like in The Society of Friends, better known as Quakers? One of the questions I asked myself before getting into the writing of this book was, 'How relevant is my Quaker experience in terms of dealing with the subject of worry and glow?'.

William Penn, the Quaker founder of the State of Pennsylvania, was by all accounts a glowing personality. Not only that, he was also responsible for one the fairest and honest land use contracts between the new settlers and the Native American People who had used the land since the dawn of time. One of the basic Quaker principles is that there is something of God/Godliness/Spirit in every human being and that is in essence what we all have in common. As a Quaker, that has been one of the driving principles for most of my adult life.

Another dominating experience was that of growing up in the middle of nature. Remo Largo a Swiss expert and author in child development often refers to the importance of small children up to the age of 5 having daily experience of nature, even if it just spending time in an urban garden or, preferably, woodland.

So, this book has been written from a very specific perspective. You, my dear reader, will be reading it from your own individual perspective with your very own life experiences. My hope is that, from time to time, during the reading of the book it rings a little bell or two in your consciousness and that you end up being a little bit enriched by the experience of reading it.

FAQ (Frequently Asked Questions) is a very useful tool for websites. However, I realised while writing this book that it is not going to be very relevant for this book because I have no way of knowing what questions, if any, my readers are going to ask.

So, rather than clutter up the book with lots of footnotes and sub-references I decided to give you my e-mail address:

mail@bryn-jones.com

Please write to me with your questions and I will do my very best to answer.

true or false?

3 WHAT IS WORRY?

Where does worry come from and what does it do to you and your body?

Let's have a look at the little boy we read about in the first two chapters. When he was born, his mother had a strong haemorrhage after the birth and had to be kept in hospital while the little baby went home. There he was lovingly looked after by his grandmother so we can assume that the stress of being removed from his mother for a few weeks was to a certain extent compensated.

Then when he was 18 months old he had a mysterious high fever and had to go to an isolation ward in the hospital for 2 whole weeks, primarily for observation. Gradually the fever went away and he could go home. But during the whole two weeks there was no human contact apart from a few minutes every day for washing and eating. Nowadays we know for certain that this was a very stressful, even traumatic, experience, but at the time, people were too concerned with the War on the one hand and on the other hand psychological research had not really done

much in this area. However a loving caring home atmosphere afterwards could well have reduced any lasting
negative effects on his development.

The year in the Sanatorium was the time when the little
boy learnt about worry. He started to worry about why he
was sent there, away from home to a room full of dying
men. Why? It was too much for the six year old and as we
now know, this was the time when he started to 'parcel'
the unpleasant experiences and began to put them away
in the darkest corners of his unconscious memory. This
is a common procedure for children as well as adults who
have undergone a traumatic experience. In practice, it
meant that when he spoke to people after he went home
he could not consciously remember any of the unpleasant
experiences and so was able to amuse the questioners by
talking about his experiences in learning English, about
the bonfire and Hitler, the oranges, American chocolate
bars and the snowball fights as well as numerous other
little pleasant incidents, all of which gave the impression
to his social environment that the year was not so bad
after all. It was just the same then as it is now; we all want
to believe that a seeming catastrophe may not be so bad
as we thought because then we don't have to have a bad
conscience. Yes, it really is often just as simple as that! Of
course it helped that through the new medication that
became available after the War, the tuberculosis could
be successfully treated so that the little boy seemed to be
quite healthy.

The tummy operation when he was 10 years old was actually an operation to remove 30 centimetres of his small
intestine because of a condition called Crohn's Disease. In
the 21st Century such illnesses are usually treated medici-
nally and surgery is the very last resort. However, that was
1948 and the parents were even warned that the little boy

had just a 50:50 chance of growing up to be a reasonably healthy adult.

We can imagine that the pain of having the metal clips removed from a particularly sensitive part of the body, the lower abdomen, was instrumental in his conscious decision to keep any suspicious signs of illness, like bodily pain, hidden from the rest of the world. No one could wish for a repeat of this tortuous medical action. Again, the 21st Century has seen enormous progress in terms of wound treatment and pain killers, not to mention increased awareness of the fact that children do feel pain, and that they do not forget, so that today there is no danger, at least in the developed world, of anyone in hospital having to undergo such an experience.

Even though it is difficult to imagine his particular experience we can, based on the description, safely assume that he had enough conscious evidence that it would be very dangerous for him to expose himself to a possible repeat of the situation. He, as a ten year old was certainly capable of devising a strategy for dealing with this danger, and he chose a combination of splitting off the painful experience (a process with which he was unconsciously familiar from his year in the Sanatorium) and consciously training himself through a form of self-hypnosis to control the expression of any reaction to pain.

One can well ask what all that has to do with worry? Even six-year-olds can worry and having to worry about the possibility of a repeat of a painful experience is certainly not a pleasant perspective. So, the six year old little boy had enough motivation to 'forget' about the pain and the ten year old was mature enough to think about a strategy to avoid having to constantly worry about going through a repeat of his awful experience. The result was that on the surface there was this ten year old bright boy with no worries and no pain.

He was very successful in hiding his pain and worries from the world. The problem was that he slowly and surely, quite unconsciously, also managed to hide them from himself. That as we shall see later, lead to more problems.

Comfort sometimes comes from situations and things we know. Like the old chair that feels good whenever we sit down in it although it doesn't exactly look like new. Or those old friends that we meet from time to time. No unpleasant surprises await us, it's comfortable. We gain comfort from the secure knowledge that things are not going to change.

Something similar takes place with old worries. They also are comfortable, if not exactly comforting. We know them and we can spend lots of time worrying about these old worries without having to worry about a new solution because we know from experience that nothing can be done about it, nothing at all. That in itself is a comfortable situation, we can lie back knowing that we can do nothing. Sometimes that is a marvellous excuse to go day dreaming.

So what does that teach us? It teaches us that we should be very attentive when we start the worry process. Are we looking for comfort or do we really want to face up to the hard work of finding a satisfactory solution to the problem?

Do ask yourself that question the next time you find yourself going into one of your old worries.

Most of us have at some point known a person for whom an empty space is something that needs to be filled. Like an empty drawer that screams to be filled up with something no matter what. Some people's minds are like that;

they are definitely not comfortable with emptiness. In fact most people are uncomfortable when their minds start to signal that it is becoming empty. You feel insecure, the emptiness seems to indicate that something dangerous is going on. It is certainly not comfortable.

This is the moment when it is easy to find something to worry about. As soon as the worrying process kicks in, the mind starts filling up and the discomfort disappears.

The significant point is that moment when we realise that the feeling of being empty is not comfortable. The problem is to be conscious of this point, because mostly it happens on a non-conscious level and we just move straight on to start worrying without even being aware that we had an opportunity to go somewhere else. Later on in this book you will be introduced to a technique for using this moment of awareness to focus on another process that involves filling the emptiness with a valuable experience as opposed to worrying.

The comfort that is involved comes not from the worrying but from the feeling that the emptiness is being filled up. We can compare it with the pleasant feeling that we get when we are able to start eating after being hungry for a while and our stomach starts to fill up after being empty. The pleasure in the mouth comes from the taste of the food, the pleasure in the stomach is due to the process of being filled up.

'It could happen', 'it should happen' or 'it will happen'. These are three common ideas that are often behind the thoughts that lead people to worry about the future, or to worry about things that may occur in the future.

Let's start off with 'could'. Where does it come from? It comes from the word 'could' that simply denotes that it is no way certain that the event will happen and that it is no way certain that the event will not happen! In other words it is a very open statement on a par with my saying that the world could end tomorrow! Who is going to prove me wrong? Tomorrow everyone can prove me wrong but today?

'Should' is somewhat different. Very often it comes along with a statement or thought, along the lines of "I really should try to stop smoking (or drinking, or .....)." The problem is that it usually ends up being an idea that fills up valuable time and space in your brain without getting anywhere except increasing your state of anxiety that you should do something but that you know damn well that you can't! Why? Because if it was possible you would have done it! So we are looking at a rather more complex issue, so rather than worrying about the 'should' it will probably be more useful to focus on the 'why', in the form of asking yourself the question 'Why should I?' That way you might end up thinking and feeling something else but hopefully it will help you get out of the vicious, endless circle of thoughts that the word 'should' tends to trap you in.

Has your dentist ever mentioned that you seem to grind your teeth at night? Well yes, some people do that and it is usually associated with worry and or anxiety. There are a lot of people around who seem to shy away from any signs of worry, people who never admit to worrying about anything. Worry is a very human mechanism. There is really no need to suppress your worry, there is no need to try to go into the world with blinkers on and try to ignore anything that could cause worry. To worry is to be human. However too much of a good thing can be bad for you. That works also for too much worry.

Let's look at the purpose of worry. Think of it as part of an 'Early Warning System.' This system works far away from our normal level of consciousness and is constantly searching our environment for signs of danger. A simple example is driving a motor vehicle. After some years experience we develop a sort of 'sixth sense' that warns us of a child on the side of the road or an approaching lorry that seems to be too fast. Many of us have experienced this kind of thing without paying too much attention to the really fantastic level of perception that is involved!

Your computer breaks down and you have to get a new one. Once the question of finance has been sorted out one would have thought that the next step, the decision about the model, would have been easy. But no, this is the point where some of us start worrying. An appropriate response would be to analyse your needs and to look for a computer that best answers those needs and then check out the best possible cost/performance factors for the individual models that are on the market. A possible last would be to let your emotions into the field and make your final decision based on how you feel when you sit before the keyboard and type something in.

There are of course people in this world for whom it is existentially necessary for them to worry at all times. No, that can't be true, did I hear you say? Yes, indeed it is sad but true. Sad because it is a neurotic malfunction that makes them worry because it stops them from looking at the other reality around them. These people, albeit unconsciously, use the time and energy involved in worry to protect them from getting involved in facing up to other issues.

If you or anyone near you falls into this category of worrying I can only recommend them to seek out a competent therapist/counsellor/analyst.

What about fantasising? Can one fantasise a worry or are there worries which are not fantasy? Do you have a great imagination? If you do then you might well be capable of imagining a horrible situation and then start worrying about the possibility of it really happening. This process starts off in a non-real, fantasy world. The situation is then projected (just like a film is projected onto the screen) into a possible future. Then your very real mind starts to worry about this completely fantasy future and then, all of a sudden, a switch takes place and the worry becomes real and the fantasy becomes a real possibility. It is after all in the future and with the sometimes amazing speeds of technological development it is often difficult to rationally predict what is going to happen in 10, 20 or 50 years. In the space of a few seconds a fantasy worry has been changed into a potentially worrying situation and then into a possible, a probable and ultimately into a concrete, real and all-consuming worry which fills up all your waking moments and even influences your dreams. That is just one of the many ways a worry starts developing a life of its own. In this book you will not only learn a bit about the various life processes that evolve around and about worry but also learn about techniques to transform these processes into somewhat more constructive channels

What has happened to the untold trenches from the First World War? Do they still remain as scars on the countryside? Have they been built over for new motorways to bring the workers, the tourists, the business people from one country of the European Union to the next? Have they been embalmed and preserved in a museum? At one time or another, all of this has happened, plus numerous other uses or abuses.

Old worries are a bit like that, it just depends on the person they belong to. Sometimes it can be of value to look back at the things you used to worry about as a child, a teenager, as a younger version of the you that you are today. Think about it. Think about all the things you used to worry about and try to figure out how it came that you don't worry about them today, or even how you still worry about quite similar issues. Try to trace back the processes involved in keeping these old worries alive rather than burying them or cremating them.

Europe and the world have changed so much since the time of the first World War, but the trenches that disrupted so many lives are still there in some form or other. Ask yourself what purposes are served by keeping your old worries alive or even what processes are involved in resurrecting some of these old worries and bringing them back to life in a new form.

Do you like James Bond? Sorry if you find this question boring or stupid, it was thrown at you just to find out if you like adventure, if you like to live an exciting life. If you are turned on by the unknown it may well be time for you to throw away your old worries and look for new ones.

If on the other hand you find peace and satisfaction in being amongst known and fixed things and situations, you might like to analyse your old worries and throw away those that are not appropriate to your current state.

Whether you are looking for new worries or doing a spring cleaning job on your old worries try to use the following questions when you are exploring the individual worry.

1. Where did it come from originally?

2. Have the original circumstances changed?

3. What were the possible benefits at the time?

4. Is this particular worry appropriate right now?

Did you understand what I was getting at with question no. 3? The question of benefits. It's an interesting topic because quite often we are motivated to worry in a particular way or about a particular thing because, quite unconsciously, we think that we will benefit. Tony was a draughtsman in a large company and would often worry about possible mistakes in his plans. He was a very experienced draughtsman and there was no objective reason for him to worry about making serious mistakes. In the cause of therapy it came out that he was desperately unhappy at his work but was shit scared of looking at other, life changing, career possibilities. His worry about making mistakes in his plans had the benefit of diverting his attention away from the much more serious question of what to do with his life.

What are the really big worries that you have? Are they life and death issues, basic human rights issues, are you worried about saying the wrong thing at the wrong place in front of the wrong people so that the secret police will come by tomorrow and bring you to a secret jail and beat you up?

Are you worried about things that are a real danger to your very existence on this earth? Do you wake up worrying where you are going to get the food for today, any kind of food at all, or where is the water going to come from to cook and drink, let alone wash.

There are today many places and people for whom these basic worries are part of their daily life. They will probably not be reading this book. There are also a few people who have had at some time or other similar experiences and who still wake up today after a particularly realistic dream and start to worry whether it wasn't perhaps a dream and that the day is going to be a hard day.

Sonia is thousands of miles away from the scene of her very bad prison experience and is living in a safe environment but still worries that something could happen and bring her back there, back to this dictatorial regime where there is, even today, hardly any security for her. She needs therapeutic support. Her worries are what I call big worries.

Well, now that we have dealt with the big worries, how about the other, everyday worries, surely they must be important. Yes of course they are important, but how much and for whom? How much energy do you waste on worrying about small things, really small things that if you really took time off to look at them very closely you will probably find out that it doesn't really matter whether you worry about them or not. But if you stopped worrying about them you would have valuable time that you could then devote to worrying about the big things.

We call that the economy of worrying. It really has do with being more aware of what you are worrying about, how important the worry is and how much time and energy you devote to the specific worry. It is only when you have some clarity about the worry that you can even begin to consider whether it is worth your while to keep on worrying about it or whether you could invest your time and energy in another direction.

Some of us have families with whom we live, others are separated from family and in some cases from friends. Just consider for a moment what the situation was like for you when you were growing up. Was your family's situation such that there was always cause for worry and concern or was it such that everything functioned perfectly and none had worries? Or something in between!

Quite often there is one single person in a family constellation that takes on the responsibility for the family or group worries. If you yourself grew up with a close emotional relationship with this person you might find yourself reacting just like her (or him) and tending to take on worries and cares that really have nothing to do with you. You might like to check them out and offer them to someone else.

The question of responsibility is an interesting one particularly in the case of an intimate relationship between two persons. A potential source of conflict is when one person worries and expects the other to do something but is afraid of being open about both the extent of the concern as well as the degree of hope that is being invested in the other person to rescue the situation. More transparency can sometimes work wonders.

Globalisation is a relatively recent word that evolved in a primarily commercial field but has in the meantime extended to such uses as the globalisation of environmental concern where groups of individuals all over the world get together to voice their concern over such issues as global changes that affect the environment.

Now looking at the difference between concern and worry we see that quite often there is a process involved that starts off with an experience which could be an oil spill, torrential flooding in summer, or a prolonged period of drought. Then a thought about the cause, and then a concern, an emotional involvement which can in turn lead either to an introverted form of worry or to some form of action.

The media is full of examples of actions so we don't have to go into detail right here. Marshall McLuhan was the first to point out such ideas as 'The Global Village' and 'the medium is the message.' I would like to now look at the idea of global worry. There is a danger that if you start to worry about how global changes affect your local environment, and do not get involved, that you could start off worrying about other, unknown, peoples and before you know it you are in a process that I would name 'the cloud of unconscious global worries.' Try to get out of that one!

The safe way is to be concerned and then start looking for other like-minded people and start planning to do something about it rather than swallowing it all yourself and ending up worrying about it.

Some years ago there was in England an organisation called 'The Flat Earth Society' and apparently there are a few people in the world that still believe that the world is flat. I can well imagine that in that kind of society there must be parents who warn their children "Don't go too far away from home otherwise you might fall over the edge of the earth and we will never see you again and that would be terrible for all concerned."

You might like to look at the various aspects of the belief systems that you were brought up within, just to see if there are still affecting the way you conduct your life. You might well find out that you have been worrying about some very irrational things and that it might well be time to throw them out.

It is a short step to worrying about sin. This is not the place to go into a theological discussion about the role of sin in the world. However there are still people who worry a lot about the effects of masturbation, ranging from going bald to even having their genitals fall off. All because they were told so by someone they believed in during childhood.

Material things are a constant cause of concern for most people on this earth. If you wake up every morning not knowing whether you are going to have anything to eat during the day or even whether you are going to have a roof over your head the next night, then it is very appropriate to be concerned.

However, the chances are that you, my dear reader, live in one of the developed societies and do not have these basic, existential concerns. But, you still worry about the possibility of such future occurrences like inflation, deflation, unemployment, wars, stock exchange, house values and so on and so forth. All quite legitimate causes for concern.

So the question is, when does a concern flip over to being a worry? Try looking very closely at your financial and material situation at this very minute and figure out how long you will be able to maintain this standard of living if one of these disasters were to take place. Then think about what you would do about it, even looking for sound advice, maybe using the Internet and if you are satisfied with the arrangements, try to decide that you will wait until it occurs and then start worrying about it. Sure, it is a superficial solution but please try it out. You may be pleasantly surprised at where your thoughts will take you when you start to look at the various solutions that crop up, provided you take your concerns seriously and really look at the various options that you will have if one these disastrous events were to affect your life.

quicksand

4 WHY WORRY?

**What are the mental and bodily
processes behind worry?**

Are you one of those who spend time living in the past, wishing for things that are long gone, missing people that you have lost touch with, not being able to correct things that you did long ago and which you now regret? Does all that sound familiar?

Living in the present is one of the most difficult tasks that we as human beings have always had to face up to. Living in the present reality has always been a problem for most human beings. Apart from, of course, special occasions like parties and holidays. Philosophers and sages all through the ages have commented on the vital importance of 'being in the here and now' in the sense of being aware and conscious of everything that is happening at the moment.

It is of course very difficult, we often feel helpless, being caught up in a treadmill with a constant drumming in the background driving us on to more and more effort.

Of course it is sometimes quite comforting to go back into our dream world of the past where even our worries have something comforting about them, where we know the themes and, of course, where we know the outcome and sometimes, the fact that there is no solution is a comfort in itself, it justifies my inactivity, my helplessness, even my self pity.

Genetic worry is not the same thing as inherited worry, it has to do with worrying about the awful things that happened in the past to members of your family. With some people the fear is so great that they end up worrying about the, usually nigh on improbable, possibility of the same things happening to them.

If you find yourself being concerned about the past lives of members of your family, try talking to your relatives about it and explore with them the possibility of history repeating itself. Of course it does sometimes happen but it is usually good to give the possibility a 'reality test' by informing yourself, in conjunction with your relatives and/or friends about the chances of it happening again in your lifetime.

If you end up being a minority of one and are still worrying about past events you should probably seriously consider counselling or psychotherapeutic help to solve your worries.

An interesting form of worry is when persons start worrying about things that happen to completely unknown persons. Fund raising projects in support of various charities often use this form of worry together with encouraging social conscience, to persuade people to donate money to the particular cause that is being promoted.

Well, you might say that with all the competition nowadays it is probably necessary and indeed acceptable to transfer money in this way from highly developed industrial consumer societies to the poor people of the world. At this point we are not going to argue with this viewpoint, rather we are going to inform you about what happens when it goes over the top.

Ann was a successful manager as well as a single parent with a five year-old son called Jimmy. She got so concerned about what was going on in some little village in the Far East that she began to neglect her son and devoted a large part of her free time to collecting money for this charity project. She actually ended up worrying so much about the charity that it disturbed her sleep and caused her to wake up from horrible nightmares. She then sought counselling and quite soon the relationship with her son became a high priority in her life and her engagement with the charity was reduced to an acceptable level.

Concern about the future of those dearest to you is central to the human condition. There is probably not a single community on earth that does not try to look after new born babies to ensure that they grow up to be healthy adults.

So when does this natural concern switch over into a non-essential worry? It is probably true to say that this phenomenon is a product of an advanced industrial way of life that puts many people under enormous pressure to spend and consume so that even though there is more than enough material wealth to go round, many people start worrying that, some day, maybe even tomorrow, something dreadful is going to happen so that they are no longer able to take care of the family.

She starts to worry that the children will not have enough warm clothes when winter comes, that her husband will lose his well-paid job, that her mother will become terminally ill. Yes, all these things could happen and they do happen every day but unfortunately it is often a reflection of too little concern about the emotional situation of the family in the present day, that is at the back of an exaggerated concern, leading on to worry about a possible material situation in the future.

When you were a child, did you get the impression that it was natural to start the day off with worrying? Some families, or at least some members of the family, deem it a matter of principle that one must start talking about their worries and worrying at the crack of dawn and never stop until they go to sleep.

The difficulty is that it tends to instil a form of mental paralysis in the children that cuts off any creative thought processes. The constant repetition of this form of behaviour means that such children grow up to be exaggeratedly concerned about such issues as job security and minimally interested in taking creative responsibility for the development of their lives.

Which is probably a good thing for a functioning state bureaucracy but not at all a good thing for the development of a national or even an individual culture.

As a conscious adult you do have the possibility of taking action against these influences, provided you are able to see clearly how they tend to control your daily life.

A completely different matter is that of families where the worries and anxieties are kept secret from the children. These children feel these worries and fears unconsciously and grow up to be adults that have difficulty in expressing and sharing their emotional life.

Worry is very much a part of a series of human emotional feelings centred around fear and anxiety.

These feelings are essential for human life because they are part of an 'early warning system' that can help us to avoid or escape from a dangerous or life-threatening situation.

Combined with a healthy instinct, it can help us avoid a potentially dangerous situation by stopping us taking a wrong step whilst climbing a mountain.

The difficulty, of course, is that we often cannot distinguish between a very real danger such as being on the edge of a precipice on a stormy night and the worrying thoughts that keep us awake at night because we are concerned about the (imaginary?) slight that we experienced during the day from a work colleague.

Both are very human. During the first part of this book we shall be exploring ways of moving away from being stuck in non-productive and non-essential worrying that use up a lot of our basic life energy that could probably be better used to enhance your daily life.

Worry is not a static process. It is not even a stable process. 'Different folks and different woes'. One could possibly say that some forms of worrying may be more useful and even more effective than others, depending on the individual person.

Let's not look so much at what you worry about, but rather at how you worry. Have you tried concentrating fully on your worry rather than let it develop its own existence whilst you are concentrating on other activities?

Do you allocate sufficient secure time and space for your worries to develop a clear cut outline or do you try to push them away into the shadow of your existence?

Can you face up to your worries or are you afraid to look at them, afraid to dig down into the different levels, the different emotional feelings, the various tastes and smells associated with your own personal worries?

Before even beginning to think about how to stop worrying, you have to get to know the particular personal processes behind the way you, yes you in person, my dear reader, have learnt to worry. As a first step, relax as much as you can, take a deep breath, look at your primary worry just now and focus on what this worry is trying to say to you. That's all, just focus and listen.

Even though the subject of worry is never taught at school the various ways of worrying or dealing with the topic of worrying, are taught, often unconsciously, in many families. What about in your family? Spend a moment thinking about it. Try to reconstruct your earliest memories of worrying, ask yourself who served as a role model and how was it that you learnt to deal or not to deal, with your worry in this particular way.

Explore the question of whether people near you spoke openly about their worries or were you left to feel and sense what they were worrying about instead and maybe even adjusted your behaviour in the hope that it would reduce their worry?

If you have children try asking yourself how you worry and if it is very different to that of your own parents and family.

Do your children know about your anxieties, cares and worries and, if not, why not?

George had a row with his girlfriend Sally, then had a bad conscience, stuffed himself with fast food, had indigestion and ended up worrying half the night that he might have a serious health problem, thus avoiding concerning himself with the more serious and real problem of his relationship with Sally.

We later found out that George often had rows with Sally, that he often felt bad afterwards, but was not capable of talking about his emotional feelings about her and the relationship.

Slowly George learnt to digest the uncomfortable emotional feelings that came up during the rows with Sally, was slowly able to talk to her about these feelings and, in time, they were even able to have a relaxed meal together after a row.

George's very real, early digestive disorder happily did not develop into any serious medical problem and his hard work on digesting his emotional problems led him to a more healthy and relaxed attitude to his nutritional as well as emotional needs.

Waiting to go into a major surgical operation theatre is one of the loneliest situations imaginable. You are completely at the mercy of a team of people who literally have your life in their hands, you will be put to sleep without knowing if you are ever going to wake up again, you are completely alone and you usually have to sign a paper agreeing that you know the high risks involved.

More than enough grounds to worry, to be anxious, to be fearful. Some people think they have to ignore their anxieties, grit their teeth, shut their eyes and just jump in there blindly.

A most interesting alternative approach was described to me some years ago by a leading heart surgeon who advised his male patients to approach it as a boxing match with death. To look at the surgical team as manager, trainer and supporting staff all of whom are dedicated to prepare and support you for the greatest fight of your life but the ultimate result is dependant on your mind, on your belief in your love of life and on your fully committed will to fight for your own life.

This was some years ago but I think that in this 21st Century he could easily extend this approach to talking to his female patients, even though, statistically speaking, the chances of having to undergo major heart surgery are still much higher if you are male rather than female.

Under what conditions do you live and work? How would you consider your living space and your working conditions: above or below average or just average? If you classified yourself as living or working in below average conditions try asking yourself who are the people who live or work below your standard. Ask yourself what they worry about and try to imagine what kind of advice you could give them on how to improve their situation, how to worry in a different way and try to address the question of whether there is any hope for them.

Hope is often missing when you get stuck in a particular worry. Some worries are like quicksand – the more you struggle to get out, the deeper you sink and the more helpless you feel.

By looking at the advice you would give to those worse off than you, you might get some clues about any possibilities of hope in your particular case. Any little bit of hope can serve as a secure stepping stone to achieve a sense of balance in your situation and then look at various possible ways out of the situation.

Life in those countries in Eastern Europe that were part of the Soviet Block was, at least for about 99% of the population, measured in terms of various shades of grey. The buildings were grey, the workplaces were grey, even people's skins often looked grey. There was very little colour and daily life reflected the grey monotony of the political structure.

Those people who grew up in such places, under a tyrannous, dictatorial regime and were not part of the political power elite, had a pretty hard time if they wanted to retain some element of self respect and not sink into a pit of apathy and despair.

Life expectancy in many parts of the former Soviet Block is still about 10 years behind Western Europe. That says much about the former regimes.

If you or any of your family grew up in one of these countries, and either succeeded to or wanted nothing more than to escape but were not able to, please pay particular attention to your prevailing worries and look for those that could reflect the fears and anxieties from that time. They do have a tendency to spread to other members of the family through both conscious and non-conscious channels. Like Martin, who kept getting nightmares about being imprisoned and tortured, that worried him during the day, until he found out that his grandfather had actually had such experiences but had forbidden his close family to talk about this period because he was so ashamed for his country, one of those smaller communist states that is still often ignored.

Some families believe in hell and terrorise their children accordingly with threats that if they do not behave, i.e. do everything their parents tell them, they would be thrown into a big fire or something similar. If you were brought up in this kind of atmosphere you could end up being worried about the consequences of some of your actions even though you consciously rejected your parents belief system a long time ago. The old unconscious memories of early childhood have a habit of influencing our grown up worries. The same principle applies to concepts of paradise, as we see from the activities of suicide bombers.

It is therefore quite useful to look at your predominant worries and from time to time check them for any unrealistic presuppositions that could influence how you react to these worries. For instance is there a tiny, little part of you that still believes that if you sin you could end up in everlasting fire? Do check all your worries regularly for signs of hidden belief systems that have remained inside your consciousness from your childhood days. They are still there, quite independent of whether your childhood memories are good or bad, many of the belief systems that you were exposed to as a child are still capable of influencing your decisions as an adult in both a positive as well as in a negative way. So, check them out!

Children often worry if they are hurt or punished, they tend to blame themselves for it and are very easily persuaded that it happened to them because they did something wrong. Some parents, even today, practice a rather horrible form of bringing up children based on fear. One of the most horrible aspects is that children are much more vulnerable than adults in this respect. They have a natural tendency to love and adore their parents and this can still be there even though the parents do terrible things to their children. Children are basically innocent and contrary to the opinion of some parents, they are not sent to this earth to terrorise their parents, they simply want love, care and attention. Nothing more and nothing less. Most children are perfectly able to understand if parents want to but are unable. They also sense if parents are really not interested and this often makes them upset, sad or even angry. This is quite understandable, if looked at from a 21st Century enlightened, educational and pedagogical perspective.

However, many adults born before 1970 in the Western part of this world suffer to some extent from this kind of upbringing, simply because it played a major role in how children were perceived at that time. The Swiss psychoanalyst Alice Miller has written extensively about the damage done to children exposed to an upbringing based on fear rather than love.

If you find yourself worrying about being punished or being hurt, try looking at your own past for signs of being controlled through threats either at home or at school or elsewhere.

What about those people who don't appear to worry at all? Do they really exist? Can one live without worrying? Everything is possible in this amazing world of ours, and of course there probably are people who live so much in the present moment that they really don't worry, but personally I like to believe that most people, men as well as women fall into the category of 'Mr Worry' from the series of children's books by the English writer Roger Hargreaves titled 'Mr Men.' In this little book Mr Worry is treated by a magician and all his worries go away. But after a week of no worries he starts to worry about why he has no worries!

However, there are some people, particularly those that have had traumatic experiences, who, in order to survive and function in the world, have repressed many of their worries and anxieties deep down into their unconscious mind and seem to function quite well without worrying. The only problem is that they often suffer from psychosomatic complaints and illnesses as a result of the unresolved conflicts raging inside them or they suffer from depression.

Mark was sexually abused as a little boy but 'forgot' all the details until he was 36 when he started getting depressed. During the analysis of his dreams many of the 'forgotten' details of the abuse came to the surface and eventually he was able to work through the various traumatic episodes, was able to mourn a part of his lost childhood and slowly opened himself to be comforted.

Why don't you stop for a minute and think about the first time you started to worry? Try to reconstruct and document the occasion and use the information to explore your own personal approach to worry.

slow

5 TIME & WORRY

**A time for worrying and
a time for not worrying.**

When is the best time to worry? Ever thought of that?
Many people start worrying when they are unable to
sleep. Others start to worry when they leave work and
some people just worry all the time. Very few people think
about consciously making time for worry. So please start
planning a time, daily, weekly or even monthly that you
will use for looking at your worries, to bring them up to
date, to analyse some of the processes that give you an uncomfortable feeling and to start worrying constructively.

One of the best kept secrets of successful worrying is to be
transparent with yourself about your worries. In this way,
particularly by applying some simple tools based on time
and motion studies, you will begin to master your worries
and stop being controlled by your worries.

Step one is getting to know your worries. You may well
think that you know them already but beware, there may
be a whole lot of other worries lurking below your daily

consciousness.

Step two involves being more efficient by focussing on the important worries.

Last but not least, step three has to do with learning how to transform a worry into a miniature dose of happiness. Remember that hit song from Bobby McFarlane, 'Don't worry, be happy'?

To worry about health is probably one of the oldest human traits. Imagine what a problem a stone age hunter would have when he woke up with a terrible fever and could not hold his bow straight. Surely he would have been worried.

In this day and age, we fortunately don't have to worry about the effects of catching a cold but we still worry about health issues. Either we are ill and worry about the development of the illness or we are not ill and worry about what would happen if we were to become ill.

We worry about the state of the health services, about all the environmental factors that could affect our health. We spend a lot of time worrying about all kinds of factors around our state of health and yet life seems to go much faster, we seem to have little time to focus on priorities or even to think about what should be a priority. Quicker, faster, more acceleration, more speed, these are the words that govern our advertising industry and that, if we are not very careful, will end up governing us.

Time spent taking care of our health is time well spent. If you find yourself worrying about your state of health, try saying STOP to yourself, spend time looking at the various factors and ask yourself "What do I really need to take care of." Then start exploring how.

Tell me, what do you do with all your time, do you use

every second to live your life fully or are you like most of us and go through life without being very aware of what we do with our time?

Some people are comfortable with time on their hands others get anxious if they have nothing to do. The problem with worries is that they crave time and attention and are always on the lookout for any spare time that's around that they can lock on to. Whether it's a big worry or any old common or garden worry makes no difference – the worry never sleeps and is always on the look out for time that it can occupy.

If you tend to worry, its quite a risky business to have too much free time, so the first thing is to check your real time table, the master time table on which you base your life and check out your life priorities, paying particular attention to any big worries and making sure that you devote an adequate amount of time to caring for the big worries, and so reduce the risk of your worries grabbing too much of your free time. Then try making a list of priorities for the really important time-consuming things in your life and compare that with how much time you actually devote to those things.

Not having enough time is a common problem for many people particularly since it seems to have become one of the modern 'civilisation diseases'. The more agricultural a society is, the more in touch is it with the time cycles and rhythms of nature and the more industrialised the society, the more it tends to be a slave to commercial time factors and schedules.

Worries tend to react accordingly – so that one often feels under pressure to get rid of the worry in the shortest possible time, to seek out some instant solution or at least a quick solution. Unfortunately our emotional feeling system does not always react in the way that our minds think it should!

Then the situation tends to become difficult; we react irritably and impatient with our immediate surroundings, dissatisfied with each and everyone that crosses our path and before we know where we are, we are in the middle of an emotional chaos and possibly forgotten what the worry was that started it all off.

One possible way out is to start to practice some form of meditation or contemplation. Don't worry at this stage about finding the best method for you, we will come back to this subject in the course of the book and you will be given some useful tips to follow up. For now, please try to adjust your mind to the possibility that a period of training in being rather than doing could be useful for you in getting out of the worry rat race.

Start off with taking a deep breath and letting it out s l o w l y. Yes, slowly letting the breath out.

How do you feel when you slow down? Do you really know what slowing down means or do you perhaps stop yourself before you get there, which is a very common reaction. Slowing down is often associated with feeling an emptiness that is very uncomfortable for most people. It involves an anxious feeling of moving into the unknown, reminiscent of childhood fears of the dark and of deep black holes.

Imagine being all alone in a cave, without light and without moving. Just being there alone, in the dark. Not being able to see but certainly able to hear, smell, taste and feel.

The chances are that even though you are not moving, your brain and thoughts are racing ahead and your imagination is starting to move into overdrive. And yet, there is nothing there except an empty cave with no light, but your creative imagination is capable of fantasising everything from a sleeping tiger who might wake up at any moment and eat you alive, to some superhero who will inject a poisonous gas into the cave, thus magically killing the tiger but saving you. I'm sure you see what I am getting at. Our unconscious mind is not a cesspit, it is a marvellous source of unbridled creative energy that can conjure up the most amazing images at a drop of a hat including ones that fill us with anxiety to the point of paralysing us. That sometimes happens when we start slowing down, so it really is no wonder that we mostly try to avoid it.

Some people go through life at a pace that leaves others breathless. Other people live at such a slow pace that it makes other people irritable and impatient.

Who becomes breathless when you live your life, you or those around you? Try considering how appropriate the speed of your particular life is for yourself; whether you are sometimes blind to the needs of those dearest to you and even whether that could mean a loss for you.

You may have noticed that if you are travelling at high speed in a car or train that there is certain loss of awareness of what is going on outside the window to your left or right but straight ahead is pretty clear. Consider whether there are times in your life when it would be useful to just stop and just experience your immediate environment including the people nearest to you.

Being and doing things very slowly can sometimes be close to passivity but if the outside temperature is approaching 40 degrees C it might be the only sane mode of behaviour.

If, on the other hand, you find yourself acting very slowly with no rational reason for it try asking yourself why you are so afraid of speed. You might find that you are spending a lot of energy just below your surface consciousness worrying about the possible results of your actions.

Meditation and contemplation have always been used as tools to discipline the mind, to help one become calm and collected whatever the surrounding circumstances.

Don't worry, this is not going to be a course in how to be a saint, I am simply going to try to introduce you to one of many mental tools that are available today.

Contemplation has always been associated with a monastic way of life, and the study of a particular theological tract or document, whereas the practice of meditation seems to me to be more useful to people living and working in the 21st Century.

There are literally hundreds of different methods and techniques for meditating so we are going to limit ourselves to giving a short description of one particular form, simply because I can talk from experience and that makes it easier for me rather than having to take someone else's experience and translate it into my own words.

This particular method is called Vipassana Meditation and is based on the technique taught by Gautama Buddha in India around 500 BC/BCE*. It involves sitting quietly paying attention to your breathing, for a period between a few minutes to around one and a half hours at a time. Then you focus on a particular part of your body, starting for example at the top of your head, then try to explore this part with all your senses, seeing it, smelling it, feeling it, hearing it, even tasting it, before going on to the adjacent section. Continue all over the body and then start all over again. It's a bit like painting the Forth Bridge, it's a never-ending task, but it is never quite the same as last time!

(BC is a predominantly Christian method of archaeological and historical dating and denotes Before Christ, whereas BCE denotes Before the Common Era).*

This is of course a very rudimentary introduction, if you like the feel of it, look for an experienced teacher in your area, the Web has enough information to help you find one.

Historical novels can make for exciting reading but can also release deep rooted worries. You may well be thinking that this is a pretty far fetched theory but please bear in mind that we are concerned here with looking at the various possible sources of worry rather than a superficial and brief look at the problem of solving how to stop worrying.

Successful novels written in a historical context often deal with traumatic experiences and if you or any member of your family experienced similar situations, reading could trigger off a chain reaction leading to a release of childhood memories that had been long forgotten.

Julia had such an experience after reading a book about Nazi Germany and suffered from night time worries and nightmares until she plucked up her courage and started to question her family. She found that an old aunt had suffered a great deal through being caught up in Poland when the Germans invaded the country during the early days of World War II. Julia's childhood fears and anxieties, after hearing about the aunt's horror stories, were buried deep down until, at the age of 40 she happened to read this novel that brought it all back with a vengeance.

Sport and worry have much in common. You can start off at any age, the earlier the better if you want to be expert, and there is no time limit on when you have to stop. There was even a documentary film published in 2010 about centenarians and world records in sport.

What denotes success? In sport, there are of course two classic standards – the one has to do with public success, with Olympic Games and World Championships; the other with personal and private success in terms of enjoyment, recreation, fitness and health.

Both demand time. So, if you are prepared to seriously tackle the question of being successful in worrying, you need to use the 'worry game technology' of H I T.

- Holistic processing.

- Involvement and commitment.

- Time.

Try to make your personal way of worrying draw on these three elements and you will soon find yourself become more efficient in your worrying and maybe begin to enjoy it.

Holistic processing means looking at the particular worry or subject from various viewpoints.

Involvement and commitment basically means taking every little detail very seriously as well as being concentrated whilst looking at your worry.

Time is the necessary glue that holds everything together.

Spontaneity spells instant danger for some people. For you also? Or are you one of those people who are very spontaneous and thus often run the risk of being labelled not very dependant because of your lively changes of direction regarding moods as well as actions and decisions.

People are different. People are difficult. Some react so quickly that others are left trying to figure out what on earth is going on anyway! It's a bit like the old parable of the tortoise and the hare. Sometimes sheer speed does not guarantee that you always win.

Similarly with worrying. Look at how quickly you tend to start worrying about something, whereas it might be more useful to spend time exploring the various available alternatives instead. For example looking at various courses of action that you could try out before getting stuck into the more passive state of worrying.

It was W.H. Davies, a 20th Century Welsh poet, who wrote a wonderful and simple poem:

'Leisure'

What is this life if, full of care,

We have no time to stand and stare?

No time to stand beneath the boughs,

And stare as long as sheep and cows;

No time to see, when woods we pass,

Where squirrels hide their nuts in grass

... ...

more at:

http://www.englishverse.com/poets/davies_william_henry

Too much worry tends to make us blind, deaf and in many ways incapable of feeling the world. Worrying can easily lead to a major loss of quality of life. That is one way of looking at W. H. Davies' poem. On the one hand it was written during the industrial revolution as the growth of consumerism took over developed societies but on the other hand it does tell us that the problem of excessive worry has been around for a long time and that it is in no way a product of a 21st Century stress-filled lifestyle.

A telescope is a very useful tool to look at potentially dangerous objects from a safe distance. Being still and quiet in a safe and protected environment, you can try raising your imaginary telescope and start looking at your real worries from a certain distance. This secure perspective can help you look at other aspects of your worries that might have escaped your attention up to now.

Do you like being early for an appointment or do you regularly turn up late, if only by a minute or two? If you are often late, that could an indication that you maybe should look at your relationship to time and caring. Try asking yourself whether you are more concerned with caring for others or is there perhaps a deep seated need to be cared for.

Maybe you were brought up in a society where being late for a date or for an appointment is nothing special, in which case you might like to ignore the above comments, although they could possibly still apply in terms of intimate relationships.

In any case the question of taking responsibility for waiting for someone or letting the person wait for you can often be a signal that it might be useful to look at your needs to control your life, even in such relative small matters as controlling the time that you meet someone else, whether an intimate friend, a member of your family or a business partner.

Time has always been associated with power and particularly with the art of warfare where there are untold examples of how correct timing influenced the battle to ensure victory or defeat. There is a wonderful story of how George Washington tricked his enemies by lighting numerous campfires and then, under the cover of darkness, moved his entire army overnight, to attack a weak position many miles away, whilst his enemy waited until daylight (because they wanted to be certain that they could be victorious) and then attacked an empty campsite!

How do you react while waiting for an appointment and it slowly becomes clear to you that it is going to be some time before it's your turn, and that means you're having to wait? Do you accept it stoically and patiently or do you get upset, angry, nervous or disappointed? Does it affect your breathing, do you feel helpless, unworthy, valueless?

Do look at your personal relationship to time and ask yourself how valuable your time is for you. If you often find yourself in situations where you have to wait, try preparing yourself for such eventualities by carrying a book to read, a notebook to make notes, a tablet or even use the time to practice meditation.

If you begin to feel nervous after a while, try to think about the possible cause of your nervousness. What do you associate with 'waiting'? Do you have any uncomfortable memories as a child of having to wait for something that turned out to be traumatic for the child. I used the words 'traumatic for the child' because there are things that happen to children which are really traumatic for them but that an adult would not necessarily find particularly difficult. For instance, the loss of a teddy bear or a pet animal. Under specific circumstances, such unconscious memories can have a powerful effect on us as adults when we have to wait for something or someone. Think about it. How do you react if you have little or no time to undertake something? Maybe you are one of those who shrug it off and say that tomorrow is another day and don't get upset about it. Or you could be one of those who immediately starts getting worried and anxious, feels worthless and incapable, feels guilty about not planning things better and so on.

Time is a very strange phenomena and has a peculiar relationship with worry. Worry has to do with future time, with an exaggerated concern for what could possibly happen in the future. If your feeling is that you are running out of time, being late for a date, having too much to do before the deadline and so on, it means that you are fast approaching the future and if you are a worry person, it means that you are fast approaching some form of disaster that you have been worrying about.

One way out of this dilemma is to picture yourself as the observer of what you are doing. Not so much observing your being but focussing on what your bodily actions are. In this way, with some practice, you will be able to step out of the vicious circle and concentrate more on being in the here and now and thus distancing your self from worry and from the possible future disaster. The chances are that you will end up in the future but still experience it as your present. Maybe even with a sigh of relief that the disaster did not take place.

Some of my readers will have seen the TV series Dr. Who. It was a very successful series with a crazy time machine that looked like an old London telephone kiosk. You might well ask, what on earth has that got to do with worrying? The answer is not a lot except that worrying can sometimes be triggered off by fantasies based on science fiction.

If you find yourself worrying about something that you saw or read about in a science fiction context you might like to consider using the same weapon to conquer the worry.

Try to imagine your very own process about getting rid of this type of worry. Don't try to forget about it otherwise you will end up like the students in a mind awareness class who were told to go a whole day without thinking about pink elephants. Of course, it is a well nigh impossible task and the task of consciously trying to stop worrying is comparable in terms of difficulty.

fear

6 PLACES & WORRIES

Are there appropriate places for worrying?

What do you think, is a doctor's waiting room a good place to worry? 'What a funny question' is a common reaction although waiting for a result of an examination is often more nerve-racking than waiting for a consultation. If I am suffering from a strong back pain, I am hoping for relief. If I have a large unexplained lump I am worried that it could be cancerous.

Usually a waiting room in a medical practice is a good place to sort out your worries, imagined or real. You will rarely be disturbed, you can be deaf to the world if you want to, and you are in a form of time capsule. You can even pretend to read.

It can be an appropriate place to prioritise your worries. To look at those worries that are particularly pressing and that are calling for action. To look at those worries that seem to be out of your control. To look at those worries that are looming just over the horizon but are as yet not identifiable.

The medical waiting room can be a useful place to start examining your own particular worries.

If you feel secure at home, then you might consider setting a particular, regular time for you to look at your worries in the security of your home environment. You can often consider various courses of action when you feel secure in yourself and that is what you will use this period of time for. You will start to explore, analyse, look at and pull apart all your worries, one at a time and look at the possible courses of action that you could try out.

Do not be concerned about whether the actions are perfect or not. The important thing is to start becoming pro-active, to do something that involves your whole attention, even to make mistakes, and to learn from the mistakes so that you can work on the next plan of action.

Loneliness is a strong and harsh enemy when it comes to going into action. Be constantly on guard that you are not being forced into inaction through the force of loneliness. Try to consider plans of action that involve you in talking to other people, known or unknown, friends or strangers. Focus on the moment, prepare the question or request well in advance, and just say it. You might well be surprised about how helpful people can be if you approach them with openness and honesty.

Worrying at work is a risky business except if your work entails working in a think-tank institute where worrying in the old sense, like a bull terrier 'worrying', i.e. chasing and attacking a bull, is part and parcel of daily work.

But since we are concerned here with emotional worrying we shall not be side-tracked and confine ourselves to apologising to those members of a think tank who inadvertently got caught up in reading this book hoping it would make their work more effective. Sorry folks!

Coming back to our main theme, even worrying at work about a work-concerned theme is a risk. Try to analyse the problem and share your perspective about possible solutions with colleagues and/or a supervisor, rather than trying to solve it on your own. Just be sure to document and file your ideas before sharing them.

Let us assume that you have a programme of to-do's for today, but you are also caught up in a big worry with no immediate way out. This is where the space principle comes in. If you have to bike up a steep hill it is almost impossible to worry at the same time, as compared to a lazy meander down a forest path. Any activity that demands a high degree of physical effort as well as concentration makes it very difficult for you to immerse yourself in your worry. There is some evidence that intense physical activity can help reduce the paralysing effect of a high level of anxiety, the main problem being how to instigate that first step towards physical activity. Just like the old adage about the main difficulty in walking 100 kilometers is that of making the very first step.

Bed is a wonderful place for some people. For others it's a torture chamber of worry that keeps them awake or drives them to seek all sorts of worries so they can sleep in relative peace.

Often the bed is the place where all the worries that have been saved up during the day are taken out and counted and worried over.

Try doing this type of work before going to bed. Look at it as a daily task like cleaning teeth that you undertake before you go to bed.

You might find that a few minutes spent ordering your worries, even making a time table of when you are going to give them your full, waking, attention in depth, will be more productive than going to bed and sleeping fitfully while trying to forget.

A park in the middle of a city is like a haven of peace in a stormy sea. It's a wonderful place to look at your worries and to list your major worries on paper or on a laptop. Go to your nearest or favourite park and recite out loud the list of your major worries – the birds and the bees won't mind and there are always corners where you can avoid other human beings if their presence makes it difficult to speak your worry list out loud. It is important to speak out loud so that your brain experiences it as coming from outside yourself. Now imagine a second person accompanying you on this walk in the park and ask her to please listen to you reciting your list of major worries and give you her feedback upon listening to you. Listen carefully and with your full attention to her (imaginary) response to your worries and you may well be surprised at what she comes up with.

Why actually go to a park or on a country walk or on the beach, you may well ask, why can't I just stay at home and do the exercise?

Well, the flowers, grass and trees of a park landscape or in any piece of open nature, give a spatial background that is the polar opposite of the confined atmosphere that prevails in any room no matter how big. These factors combine to release parts of your emotional fantasy life when you are in a park that would not necessarily come out if you stayed at home. Try it out. Spending time outdoors will in any case be good for your breathing and as you will find out later, deep breathing is beneficial for the transformation of worrying into glowing.

One of the nice things about living in a city is that you can choose your identity. You can choose to be anonymous in this huge mass of people or you can try out various new identities without fear of being ridiculed or laughed at by friends, relatives or acquaintances. You can also experiment with expressing some of the emotional feelings that you have difficulty letting out.

You can for instance go to a dark cinema and cry your heart out without having to answer awkward questions afterwards. Some cinemas even have double seats where couples can be even closer together, but the darkness can also be a protection for lonely and worried singles, a place to face their deepest and darkest worries but still get a feeling of being safely anonymous in the protective security of a cinema audience.

You can even push your way through a crowd and experience the closeness, the intimacy of other physical bodies without having to ask permission or having to worry about being rejected if you did ask. You can relax and bathe in the warmth of a crowd, whether in a department store at sale time, in a busy shopping street, a theatre bar during the interval or even at a football match. They are all good places to try out different approaches to confronting your worries related to closeness to other human beings. Two of the most basic human anxieties are those associated with the fear of being in a confined space on the one hand and the fear of falling into endless space on the other.

Darkness in a cinema or a theatre can be a source of comfort and safety as opposed to a dark night in the country, particularly for town dwellers. When we feel safe from outside danger it is somewhat easier for us to look at our inner feelings and begin the process of looking at and analysing our deepest worries. In this respect our stomach can be useful because it tends to go tight when we confront some of our deepest worries and that is a sign that it is worthwhile to explore further. Try locating the particular emotional feeling that is uppermost when you approach the worry and save it for afterwards when you can look at it in peace and quiet, in the light, and possibly use paper and pen or a computer to explore further.

Some people use the Internet as a form of sleeping pill, others to escape from their own personal reality and some try to get away from their worries by watching TV.

Why not try using your computer to consciously inform yourself about the things that you worry about rather than using it to divert your mind from your worries.

You may not be able to stop worrying about a specific subject but you can at least inform yourself fully.

'Home is where the hearth is' is an old English saying. It is often also the place where conflicts are. It is a very unusual family that does not have conflicts of one form or another. Either they are openly discussed or they are more or less discreetly put away. In any case, there is usually at least one member of the family who suffers from the fact that the conflict is not openly addressed.

If you yourself are one of the sufferers of an unresolved conflict that keeps you worrying about it, the first step is to try to bring it out into the open. The next step is to ensure a situation where 'eye-level communication' can take place. That means that each member has equal rights of expression and that any hierarchical pyramid of power does not apply during the discussion. That is of course difficult in some families!

But lets assume that the participants agree to give it a try. Next step is to establish if there is a particular one-to-one conflict. If so, it might be a good idea for these two to agree to meet up without the others. In this one-to-one meeting agree that each person can talk without being interrupted for 5 minutes; then the other. Try to talk from a 'me' perspective rather than being the accuser. Try saying 'I worry a lot about...' rather than 'You always treat...'. The final 5 minutes is time to exchange views. It is important that the participants have the same amount of time even though part of it is used in silence. Try it, it sometimes can be very effective.

Holidays are a tricky subject; they are designed to be a time for re-creation for renewal and rest. Often they turn out to be full of stress, conflict and worries.

Experience shows that holidays where one partakes in physical and bodily activities that are in sharp contrast to one's daily life activities, have a higher chance of working as a refreshing break.

This is one more example of how body and mind really form a unit that can work positively in such circumstances, where life energy is used in an unaccustomed way, thus diverting energy from being spent worrying.

A relaxed body makes it much easier for the mind to concentrate on the present moment and if the setting of the holiday is strange or new, that could well lead to interesting observations, thoughts and even emotional feelings.

Friends can often help when it comes to moral and emotional support when your worries tend to be too much. They can also be an excellent source of creative ideas for possible solutions if your worries can be formulated as such.

The formulation or expression of worry is an important and valuable subject in itself. If you are prone to worry about something that is in itself somewhat foggy or misty you run the risk of getting bogged down in the worry in the same way as it is risky to walk through marshy ground when it is dark.

Choose a friend with care and try to put your worry into words that are understandable. Once you have defined the problem it will be possible to start looking for a solution, otherwise you will end up like the tourist car driver lost in the lanes of western Ireland in the 1960s who asked a local how to get to Dublin and was given the reply "Oh dear, if I ever wanted to drive to Dublin I would never start from here!".

So the first step is to really look hard at your worry, try to write it down, speak it out loud if only to yourself and try to locate the primary problem that is behind the worry particularly if you have the feeling that you are bogged down. Then, choose a friend or friends with care and share the problem with them and ask for their ideas on how to solve it.

If you find yourself at the moment without any friends, try to imagine a friend that you would like to have and go through the whole procedure with this imaginary friend. You might be surprised at what comes up.

Sharing your worries with strangers can be a very exciting adventure even though a bit risky! It might be better to start off in the third person, that is by describing the 'worrier' as if she was a friend of yours. That can help you keep a certain emotional distance from the problem and help you to really listen to what the stranger has to say about it.

You never know what could come up. Stephen was travelling by train one day on his way to visit his favourite uncle and was worried about telling him that he was in financial trouble through a failed business idea. Travelling opposite him was a very sympathetic fellow who turned out to be a business manager on the way to some conference or other and they started talking. At some point Stephen started talking about his fictitious 'friend' and his friend's uncle, and the stranger started to make some very pertinent remarks about the failed business. They were so very much to the point that Stephen started to seriously explore the possibility of starting all over but from a different perspective.

Arriving at his uncle's place Stephen explained the whole situation including a possible new start and his uncle agreed to help him financially for a few months and within three years the new business was on its feet and Stephen could repay his uncle. He never did see the stranger again but is still thankful for his timely advice.

We have been looking at what happened to Stephen during his train journey. Of course it does not always happen that you have an interesting stranger opposite you!

A journey, whether by train, bus or car can be a useful way to look at your worries, to sort them out, bring them up to date or even throw them out. Driving a car is another matter and focussing on worries could lead to an accident so it is not to be recommended, but being a passenger in a car is OK.

Try planning how to approach your worries. Look for a common structure in your worries and especially look at what sort of 'life goals' would help you to live with your worries, even though they do not go away.

Listed below are the sort of questions that a long journey particularly on your own, is especially good for.

+ Where does my worry come from?

+ What could it lead to if the worry turns out to be reality?

+ What action could prevent the worry escalating?

+ What can I do to foster this kind of action?

+ What would happen if the worry turned out to be false?

Being lonely and also worrying is not very pleasant. Sometimes however it is necessary to be alone in order to look behind the worry for the emotional feelings that are often hidden there.

Consciously going out into nature, even climbing hills or mountains is quite a good idea to create some distance from your fellow beings. Then you can sit down, be quiet, start going down inside yourself, to your belly and look for the hidden emotional feelings that are bound to be there. After a while you will be able to sense some movement and by being patient, very patient, you will begin to feel.

Basic and universal human emotions are:

fear, anger, disgust, sadness, joy and surprise.

Take your time and see if you can feel even just a little bit of one or more of these emotions inside you. Then try being very caring towards yourself and allow the feeling to grow just enough so you can recognise it for what it is.

Don't be surprised if your body begins to express itself before your mind can grasp what is happening!

Once you have began the process of isolating your emotional feelings you can begin the process of researching how the feeling relates to your worry.

Now you can practise the SLOB technique:

S stop

L look and listen and

O open your

B belly

burn

7 WHO'S WORRIED?

About the different types of people who worry.

Did you ever think about what Father Christmas worries about? Increasing earth population, climate change, negative birth rate amongst Germans, change in the earth's magnetic field; surely there is a lot that he could worry about.

But, he doesn't! He just keeps on going about his task year after year after year, just delivering the gifts to the kids.

Father Christmas, Santa Claus or whatever his name is in the various cultures, is mostly pictured as being fat or rotund and is usually jolly and happy and oozes comfort and warmth.

Does that mean fat people don't worry? No, it doesn't. It does mean however that sometimes fat people are insulated from their worries as if the body mass tends to either focus their attention on their being fat, in which case they worry about being fat, or the body mass makes it difficult for them to sense certain body reactions that could trigger off fear or anxiety. It all adds up to give the impression that they are a steady source of comfort and stability, which in turn is not compatible with a person who worries.

So, if you are overweight or even if you think that you are fat, look at yourself to see if you worry. If you worry, then please read on. If you do not worry try asking yourself why you are reading this book. It could well be that a not very conscious part of you has some hidden worries and wants you to pay some attention to them.

Scrooge, a mean character from the novel 'A Christmas Carol' by Charles Dickens is always pictured as a thin man. Why is that? Why are thin people often associated with being mean and stingy? Do people think that they try to save on food or that they are being punished by the gods for being mean? Whatever, all over the world, mean people are always pictured as being thin!

People in prison are usually thin because they do not get enough to eat or just about enough to survive and so it is understandable that we tend to associate thin people as being punished.

A phenomena which is also associated with being thin is the fashion industry, particularly the models even though there does slowly appear to be a trend towards more flesh. Possibly allied to that is the tendency amongst young girls to 'anorexia' and 'bulimia' where they either do not eat or eat and then deliberately vomit the food. All, just to be thin. We can, at least in these cases, be justified in thinking that there are elements of both punishment as well as being mean to themselves in these actions.

If you are thin or even if you think that you are thin do please consider the above, particularly if you consider yourself as a person who does not worry very much.

All kinds of people worry and all kinds of people do not worry. Intelligent people are not always very intelligent when we look at the content of their worries! They sometimes worry, without any real need, about small and relatively unimportant matters. But don't we all if looked at from afar!

That is always fascinating about other people's worries. From a certain distance we can see that the chances of the worry being converted into reality are extremely low but if we are in the middle of a worry we are often convinced that it will almost certainly take place.

If we were able to travel at the speed of light we might be able to get so close to the time of the event that we are worrying about that we might be able to see it. We might also be able to see that there is not the remotest chance of it really happening. Intelligence might well be very useful for solving problems with a high logical and rational content but most worries and, in fact, most unconscious processes are products of irrational constructions and processes.

That does not mean that you have to be stupid to not worry, but it does mean that you have to learn how to be emotionally intelligent if you want to get to know your worries.

What exactly is emotional intelligence? It has do with knowing about your emotional feelings and, according to some, has to do with your self-perceived ability to also control your emotional reaction to life situations.

It can be learned, but it is normally not a part of a school curriculum. So how do you learn to be emotionally intelligent?

Let's start off by asking yourself how you score in the following categories....

Adaptability: flexible and willing to adapt to new conditions.

Assertiveness: forthright, frank, and willing to stand up for your rights.

Emotional perception (self and others): clear about your own and other people's feelings.

Emotional expression: capable of communicating your feelings to others.

Emotional management (others): capable of influencing other people's feelings (this is of course a tricky one).

Emotional regulation: capable of controlling your emotions.

Impulsiveness (low): reflective and less likely to give in to your urges.

Relationships: capable of having fulfilling personal relationships (another tricky one!).

Self-esteem: successful and self-confident.

Self-motivation: driven and unlikely to give up in the face of adversity.

Social awareness: accomplished networker with excellent social skills.

Stress management: capable of withstanding pressure and regulating stress.

Empathy: capable of taking someone else's perspective.

Happiness: cheerful and satisfied with your life.

Optimism: confident and likely to "look on the bright side" of life.

What about people who work primarily with their hands? It really does not seem to matter a great deal when it comes to worrying. History professors as well as plumbers both have the capacity to worry. The deciding factor when it comes to dealing with their worries as well as the anxieties that often accompany them, lies in how developed their 'emotional intelligence' is. It really does seem to play a very important role in how they deal with their worries.

Theodor was a renowned European expert in some little known aspect of economics. Very clever, very successful as an academic but constantly worried about having to go to hospital. Guess what? Yes he did have to go one day, the tests showed he was OK and he then started to worry about what if the tests were wrong.

After learning some more about developing his skills in relationship to his own emotions he was slowly able to understand the processes behind his worrying and learnt to give them their proper and appropriate place and time in his life.

People who work on a production line in an industrial factory have some concerns that are directly connected with their work. Issues such as the increasing use of automation making workplaces redundant, changes in the market making the whole factory redundant or even pressure to reduce job security. All these factors can combine to induce great concern that can lead to constant worrying that in itself often leads to lack of concentration at work that then ends up in loss of the workplace.

A very difficult situation that has lead some European Trade Unions to call for psychological counselling at the place of work.

Office workers have their own specific concerns. Mobbing and Burn-Outs are two major issues in the 21st century.

Mobbing can not only lead to extensive worry, it can escalate into anxiety and even clinical depression.

'Burn-out' first arose as a clinical issue in the 1990s amongst social workers, where the constant stress, particularly amongst street workers was beginning to take its toll and leading to staff having to take time off to recover, leading to more stress amongst the remaining staff, and so on. A particularly vicious circle.

Meanwhile the syndrome has moved into the commercial and administrative world with economic and financial factors playing an important role so that all kinds of people are now suffering, from office clerks to high level managers.

Mobbing as well as Burn-Out are beyond the scope of this book. If you are concerned that they might apply to you or someone dear to you, do please seek psychological advice, the sooner the better.

It is no way certain that people who work long hours indoors, particularly in an air-conditioned environment worry more than the average, but it is certain that many air conditioning systems are antiquated or are not serviced regularly and that often leads to colds, lack of concentration, etc. which can then lead to warnings at work, leading eventually to being worried about either losing the job or worrying about having to change jobs.

Health is a major factor in indoor working environments and progressive companies are well aware of it. But we all know that there are a number of not very progressive companies out there and to work for them does increase the risk of worrying.

Some offices and workshops/laboratories, with the exception of the high-tech ones, (where the air conditioning is usually first class – not always because of the people but because of the processes!) are like cages with a high-risk, non-healthy climate. What to do? There are two major factors that can increase your resistance to common illnesses: exercise and nutrition. Try to work out often and try taking a fruit or vegetable juice day once a week. Just drink juices all day long, no solids, no coffee, no smoking. Just try it and do it!

But, you may say, what about people who work out-doors? People working on building construction, farm-ing, fishing, surveying and so on. Charles is an organic farmer and was constantly plagued by worries; would the weather turn before the crop was in, would he get enough seasonal helpers, etc. The list was never-ending until he changed two things. Firstly, he began a daily routine going out alone on his mountain bike which slowly and surely brought his heart and blood circulation into a healthy state, and then changed his eating habits and ate much more of his tasty produce in a raw, uncooked state.

Did that mean that he stopped worrying? Not at all, but it did mean that he was much calmer and that the level of worry was brought down so that it did not interfere with his daily work routine and did not keep him awake at night. It was a 'management success'.

Traditional work like farming and fishing are usually a long way from the romantic way of life that people from cities are often brought up with. Global industrialisation has long caught up with agriculture and fishing with mechanised harvesting picking up tons of vegetables a day and automatically loading them on special transport; at the same time they leave un-picked vegetables on the ground which stay there and rot, because it is not eco-nomically viable to send people in to clear the ground! 50 kilometres away people are having to go to charity kitchens to get enough food! Food has become an industrial product.

There are 'roots for food' movement based on scavenging. People in highly industrial societies are starting to organise troops to gather foodstuffs from supermarkets, farmers markets, even factory farms. These foodstuffs have either been thrown away as garbage because the 'best by' date has gone by for 2 hours or because it is uneconomical to harvest or store. We are not talking about a few kilos. Estimates range from 100 to 300 tons of thrown away foodstuffs in the USA per DAY. In early summer 2014, the EU started to consider abolishing expiry dates on pasta, simply because its not relevant but also because they realised that every year tons of pasta were being thrown away because of the date! Now that really is something to laugh about and to worry about.

As one gets older one becomes more fragile. For many people, that leads automatically to being more worried about accidents and illnesses. Advertising for the major pharmaceutical industry plays on these worries to persuade people to buy 'just in case' without always being very transparent about the risks involved.

Many elderly people turn to religion for comfort and solace, often because of worries about death and what is going to happen afterwards. Those who have been subjected in their childhood to sermons about the horrors of hell are likely to be plagued by worries influenced by such pictures.

Having to be dependant on others, whether paid professionals, family and relatives or even the state is a major source of worry amongst the senior citizens of the Western world as well as to an increasing amount of people in the Eastern world.

What to do about such worries? The internet, the web, social networking or any other words that you may use for online services, are a truly marvellous way of getting information about how to get out of a purely passive, worried and anxious state of mind. We have to get back to basics like exercise and nutrition. Try googling around until you find an exercise plan that suits you, visit your local fitness centre, join a local sports club, go for power walks every day, get a bike and use it; the list is endless. And so is the list of excuses! It's the same with food and a nutrition plan. The world is full of useful information on how to feed yourself healthily. Too much information, so that many people get confused and end up feeling helpless and incapable and simply do nothing.

Children don't worry? Of course they do, but as an adult it can often pay dividends to work at being younger. Not necessarily to be more childish but maybe a little more child-like in terms of getting joy and pleasure out of life. Your body will be thankful for the loving attention and your mind will be helped to be more flexible and open. All kinds of activity in the areas of sport, fitness and wellness can help make you feel younger than your biological age and lead to a more carefree attitude to life, which in turn can lead to higher resistance to common ailments.

Flexibility gets harder as one gets older. We all know people who start early with the process of hardening not just of the arteries but also of the mind. Even mainstream thinking is now slowly recommending physical health as one of the bits and pieces of the process of staying mentally flexible and open.

One day of fasting per week is a great way of training you to be open to the riches that can be gained by going against the stream of consumerism. Just imagine what an effect it would have on the world if everyone in the so-called 'first world', the world of industry, commerce and above all consumerism, would take one day off from all the consumer products of the food industry. What a revolution!

It reminds me of the general increase in health amongst the populace of Great Britain during the second world war as rationing was introduced. One of the main health hazards in present-day Germany are 'Civilisation Diseases' caused by an over-consumption of industrialised food-stuffs.

Mars was the Roman god of war and the lover of Venus, the goddess of femininity and love and this dichotomy has influenced Western culture since then. However other cultures have different mythologies and different gods!

There is very little evidence that women or men worry in a different way.

But it is certain that different cultures have different ways of worrying or at least they have different sense of values when it comes to determining how important the worry is. Just imagine the different possible reactions if a little girl in a poor village in north east India worries because she does not have a computer. The chances are that some of her compatriots would sympathise and that at least one of her grandparents would not be able to understand her concern, and possibly try to ridicule such notions.

Lets look at two major modern myths. The one is that all Westerners life a life of luxury and the other is that all people from the East know how to meditate.

But there are some differences between East and West apart from geography. There is certainly a long tradition of meditation in the east, particularly in the Buddhist influenced cultures but even there it was only a minority who practised, just like in the West there have always been contemplative monastic orders, but only a small minority lived like that.

Even a monastic life is no safeguard from worrying; many years ago at a large Buddhist monastery in Sri Lanka I got to know some monks who were really quite agitated and worried about the possibility of violent revolutionary activities destroying their way of life. This was just before the Tamil Tigers demonstrated that their anxieties were justified.

However there is certainly at least one form of meditation that I can talk about from personal experience that can be valuable as a tool for containing your personal worries. This is, according to some sources, the form of meditation that Buddha himself taught his closest followers – monks like himself. It is called Vipassana Meditation and there are numerous teachers and teaching centres all over the world.

There is certainly no doubt amongst most 21st Century social, psychological and medical observers that increased industrialisation brings with it an increase in anxiety-producing lifestyles.

It is when we look at the solutions proposed that we come across divergences. Some look at the means of production; some look at a perceived moral decline in society and still others look at seemingly insufficient laws and regulations around matters concerning national security.

Put any number of sociologists, psychoanalysts and politicians in the same room and you will find that number of possible causes and at least that same number of possible solutions.

You have probably realised by now that the basic problem of worry is not going to go away. Human beings are probably always going to be prone to worry. You and me included!

The good news is that there are quite a lot of actions that you can undertake to keep the your worries at an acceptable level, so that they do not escalate too far into life-energy-sapping anxieties.

How about starting off with learning how to be efficient at worrying!

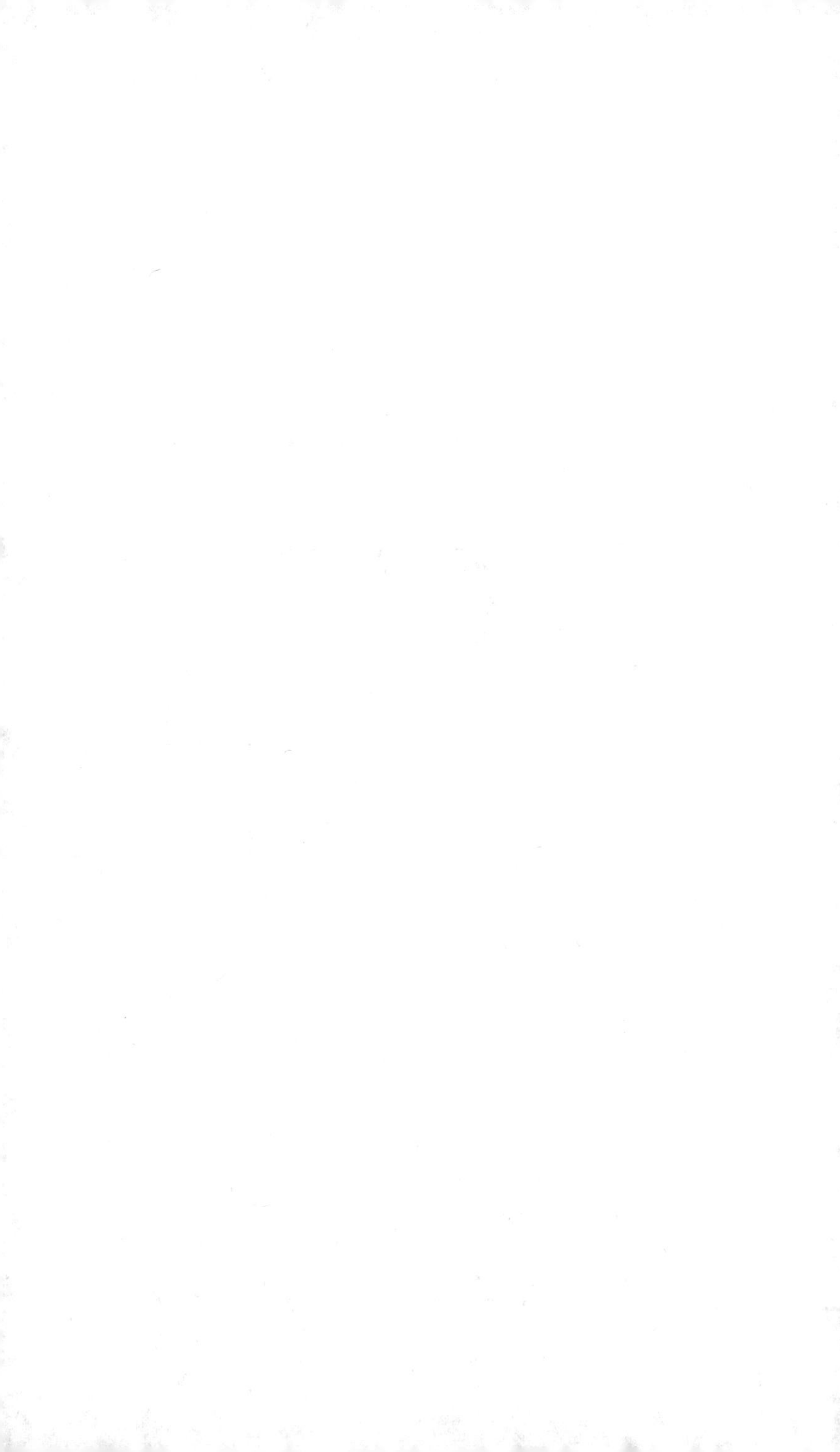

now

8 WORRY EFFECTIVELY!

Appropriate ways to worry.

Stop. Stop reading, stop thinking, stop doing whatever you are doing or even thinking of doing and just breathe. Yes, just consciously take in a breath of air, taste it, feel it, let it slowly go into your chest and even into your belly and then ask yourself the following question:

What am I really worried about right now?

Digest and remember the answer, let your breath out if you haven't done so already and write down the answer to your question.

Do that three times and you have a good foundation for establishing a triangle of priorities of worries that you can work on.

If the answers you got were too chaotic, complicated or in

some way difficult to express, go through the whole process again until you find three worries that you can write down in a form that is understandable for you.

You will now learn a different way of approaching your worries.

Worries are very sensitive things. They demand a lot of attention all of the time. Try thinking of them as little children in a supermarket who start crying when the mother is shopping. Some mothers stop shopping, turn to the child, feed it or cuddle it or whatever and the child is happy and the mother can carry on shopping. Other mothers start slapping, shouting, get angry and the whole shop gets involved and the situation escalates and nobody is content. The mother is angry, the child still cries, other customers get annoyed or go away and the cash desk slows down!

So, the first thing is to look at your worries and not ignore them.

You may well be thinking 'what's all this about how to worry, what is wrong with the way I have been worrying up to now, it seems to work all right; anyway I don't really want to worry, I want to stop worrying!'

That's ok, the only problem is that worrying is a very basic human function that will not go away! The secret is to keep it at a useful level and not let it escalate into anxiety and fear, which could possibly then lead to definite negative influences on your daily life.

So please try to look at your present way of worrying in the same way that you look at your attic or cellar; is it full of things that you haven't used for years and that you will probably never use, is it full of cobwebs and musty smells, does it reflect some childish traits left over from long ago, or do you just worry because it is an honoured tradition in your family to worry in this way.

What is so very special about your old way of worrying? What benefits do you get from worrying this way? If you are still convinced that you don't need to change how you worry, just skip the rest of this chapter and look at the rest of the book.

How different are your worries now compared to when you were young? And how different is your way of worrying compared to then? Try looking at the way you worry to ascertain if you tend to worry more about what could happen to you or is it more centred on persons or things outside you. Whether your 'worry environment' is local or global, meaning whether your external worries are more concerned with worrying about family and friends and your local neighbourhood or more concerned with foreign peoples or countries or even with worrying about something that happened in or from outer space.

Babies get anxious when they don't have enough to eat, when they don't have enough human contact, or when they are forbidden or punished for exploring their own bodies. Many adults are also concerned about these basic issues but normally in our western or western influenced civilised society these basic anxieties have been drilled out of us or, in other words, pushed into the non-conscious realm of our being. During the course of psychotherapeutic treatment they often come into awareness and the process of integrating the knowledge into daily life is often hard work and takes time.

Try looking at your worries from such a perspective and if you think some of the ideas mentioned above apply to you personally, don't hesitate to seek adequate professional help to deal with any difficulties that may arise.

One of the difficult issues around worrying is that it has to do with the future, never with the present. Even though it is often based on past experiences or memories, the worry always concentrates on what could happen in the future, if this or that would take place or if I do this or that or even I do not do this or that. Worrying is a cyclical process – it keeps going around in circles with no apparent way out.

Stop. Stop breathing, stop thinking, stop doing. Just for a minute. You don't have to worry about getting stuck, you will soon start breathing, thinking and doing. But if you just concentrate on how the breath comes in and out, if you can distance yourself from your thoughts and just observe your thoughts and if you can just sit quietly without moving, well then you have just taken the first step towards a new way of worrying. You have taken the first step towards conscious worrying.

The concept of constantly trying to live in the present, or in the here and now, is not a new concept, it keeps on coming up in such varied fields as break dancing, acrobatics, trapeze artistry, Jungian psychoanalysis, Eastern philosophy, yoga, meditation and the Esalen influenced humanistic psychologies of the 1960s.

Whatever way, method or technique you personally choose to start living more in the present moment, you will certainly notice that it will affect your way of worrying in a positive way. When you start applying the principle of here and now to your way of life you will also start on the path of making your worries a more effective and constructive part of your daily life rather than leading to a loss of energy and joy.

Worry has basically got to do with the future. Even though you, as the worrier, use your experiences or your imagination or your emotional feelings from the past or even from the present, as the foundation on which you build your worries, the worries themselves have to do with what could happen in the future, whether that future is in an hour or even in a year. What you, as maybe all of us, often forget is the question mark that is always there. It is not at all certain that it will happen – we worry about the possibility that it could happen and ignore the fact that it is 'only' a possibility and not a certainty. That is why you keep reading about the importance of being in the present time. I can't emphasise enough that the question of time is essential to the whole topic of worrying. It sounds simple but is very hard indeed to practice being in the present time for more than a few micro-seconds.

Charlie was always worried about being ill in a foreign country and avoided going abroad on holiday for many years. Then he changed his job and had to go to India for some months. You can imagine how he spent hours getting medical insurance and prophylactic medicines for just about everything before stepping on to the plane. Well he did get to India, he found his work there very reward-ing, did not get ill but, one day he lost his passport. Being an efficient manager he was not fazed but fought his way through both the Indian and his own bureaucratic jungles and eventually got a new passport. The significance of this story is that he later realised that through his concentrated attention on solving the problem of the lost passport he completely stopped worrying about his becoming ill. This experience was central to his later motivation to profit from psychotherapy on his path towards freeing himself from excessive worry.

Please note that this book is designed to give some infor-mation about the very basic human condition of worry. It is not at all a substitute for professional therapy or coun-selling.

In 2010 the German public, according to the medical insurance organisations, suffered more from mental disturbances than in previous years. Of course, there was a debate about whether it was really so, or was it because the insurance companies paid for you to visit a psychotherapist without making such a big fuss about it, as compared to 10 years ago.

The experts continue to debate whether there is really an increase in mental disturbances or whether society has simply become more open to the idea that treating mental disturbances really should not carry more stigma to it than going to the dentist. There will probably always be people who are afraid to go to the dentist and there will probably always be people who are more afraid to look at their anxieties rather than looking for a sympathetic psychotherapist.

Worry is always real. Always. It is very real in the sense that it has a very real impact on the life of the worrier. However, the background, the underlying causes for the particular worry are not necessarily 'real' in the sense that they are certain to lead to the future catastrophe that the worry is based on. Just like a conscientious gardener, we have to constantly check that the undesirable 'weeds' don't take over and choke our garden to death, i.e. that our worries do not restrict our basic life force. Just like there are fashions in gardening, there are themes to worry about that are more attractive for some societies than others. I'm thinking for instance about ecology, a theme that is of interest for many in Germany and the U.K., but is more or less ignored by 98.5% (based on the voter turn-out for the fledgling Green Party, in 2008, the only party to mention this theme), of the people in Bulgaria!

Does it help to say to someone who worries 'Oh, don't worry about it, it's just a fantasy, a product of your creative imagination'? Not really, whether the worry is based on a misinterpretation of some facts or based on a dream or a fantasy, for the worrier, the emotional part of the worrying, the feelings that can sometimes paralyse one for a long time, these feelings are very, very real.

One of the interesting characteristics of emotional feelings is that they grow from inattention. Yes indeed, emotional feelings gather strength from being left alone. Just as certain that fruit mixed with sugar in a glass bottle and left alone in the sun will slowly turn into a strong alcoholic liquor, so can emotional feelings ferment inside a human being and suddenly express themselves and surprise everyone including the person in who's being the feelings grew.

That is why we keep coming back to the importance of paying attention to your worries, paying concentrated attention, as if your very life depends on it. A future, more or less, peaceful life may well depend on the attention you give to your emotional feelings, so maybe you should start right now.

What about worrying about things that are really possible? Things like environmental catastrophes like leaking oil wells or natural catastrophes like tsunamis. Susie, a Bulgarian who emigrated to the USA and who returned to Bulgaria after 2007, told me that for her personally, the biggest difference was that if they saw something that was a problem, the Americans immediately thought about what they could do to alleviate the situation; the Bulgarians started to complain.

Maybe there are two main types of worriers, the ones who analyse their worry and start making plans, even plan A and plan B and start going into action, whereas the other type lets the worry take over and slowly find themselves being in paralysis and unable to think clearly.

After reading this book you won't have any more excuses as to why you end up being a slave of your worries! You have to start right now by looking at your worries, analyse your worries, even label them in terms of local/global; fantasy/real possibility; big/small, etc. You've probably got the idea by now. However the main thing is to go onto action and start doing something rather than just sitting there and worrying! If you work primarily with your head or mind or brain, in other words not primarily with your hands and your physical being, try doing some work with your hands when your worries start to get you down. Even washing up by hand, if you're not used to it, can be quite challenging and can sometimes divert your consciousness into a more present day direction.

We have just been looking at things that could possibly happen. Now lets look at things that have a high probability of happening. Jenny was worrying about how she could pay the mortgage on the house after her husband went off with someone else. This worry was justified on the grounds that the bank had said that they would foreclose if she did not come up with the money. The first thing to do in such a situation is to plan a strategy for a way out. In Jenny's case it meant immediately letting a couple of rooms to other people in order to increase her cash flow to pay the mortgage and to give her breathing space to come up with a long term strategy. So its important to assess how high is the probability of the 'worst possible case' happening, make a list of priorities and then take some difficult decisions, but take them anyway, firstly on a short term basis to move out of the emergency situation and then, in peace and quiet, look for a long term strategy to deal with the situation. In any case it calls for good management of the situation and it may be useful to draw on the source of the verb 'to manage' for some useful clues. It seems that the origin of the word is probably from the 16th Century 'maneggiare' in the sense of being able to handle a team of horses. Just imagine how difficult it must be if each horse has its own idea of which way to go!

How is it that some people are constantly worrying about things that can't possible happen, about situations that are really impossible? One way of looking at this problem is to take a look at the various theories about the non-conscious part of our consciousness. Sigmund Freud was the first to codify the various levels of consciousness and of course there have been countless theories that have sometimes built on Freud's foundation or even created another foundation. In any case one common factor that constantly occurs when we look at the unconscious mind is that the processes that take place there do not follow the rules of logical thinking that we are accustomed to. Who has not, at one time or another at least, heard of someone flying in a dream? Impossible? Not in a dream! So if we assume that worries draw upon the unconscious mind for their material, just like dreams do, then it begins to make some kind of sense that worries could well be based on things that are 'impossible'. In my experience one of the most effective ways of dealing with this form of constant high-level worry is through a psychotherapy based on depth psychology. Whether the orientation of the therapist is more Freudian or more Jungian or even a different system, does not really matter – what is important is that the client and the therapist get on with one another.

When I was at school one of the most horrifying images was of the 'Black Hole of Calcutta', a prison in the old Fort William, Calcutta, India where apparently (modern historians tend to think that the account was exaggerated) 123 prisoners died out of 146 prisoners held in a room measuring about 4.5 x 5.5 metres. It was vividly portrayed by our history teacher as an example of how horrible human beings can be to each other. I am mentioning this because you will notice that if you concentrate on the feeling inside you if you read the above once again, slowly, you may well get the sense of helplessness that emerges when imagining oneself in a tight space, in the dark, with far too many other people. That is why worrying alone at night is so distressing, because of the accompanying feelings of helplessness. The best way out is to get up and do something. What you do is secondary – whether it is conscious work on your mind like mediation or contemplation, writing a diary/journal or building a model aeroplane, the important thing is not to be enslaved by the worry. And please don't start now worrying about the loss of sleep ... your body will soon recuperate after a worry-free bout of sleeping.

We have looked above at the problems associated with worrying at night, let's now look at worrying during the daytime. Most people, particularly those who have been brought up in an urban environment, have a pretty good idea of what it means to be afraid of the dark or in the dark, and thus can really understand what a problem it is to worry at night. Worry during the day, on the other hand, is something that most people get taught. Who has not been told as a teenager: 'It's time you started to worry about your future!'. In other words, a major part of education is still based on teaching children at a very early age to start worrying, about punishment, about winning, about exams, and so on and so forth. So we can assume that you, the reader, are an expert in worrying. We are not going to even try to stop you from worrying (surprise, surprise!), but we hope to help you change both the quality and the quantity of your worries. The first thing is to make a schedule, a timetable, with enough space and time for you to devote every day to worrying. Strange idea? Try allocating 15 minutes every day to make a list of your worries and then list them in order of priority, the most important ones being labelled with an A or with a 1 and so on. Once you have made the list, try devoting the next 15 minutes period (some people make the list in one session, others need days or weeks to make the priority list) to really looking at the high priority worry, feel the emotion within it, explore the worry and get to know the worry. Then go on to the next on the list, until you have worked through all the worries on the list. Then make a completely new list. You may well be surprised. But please don't stop the process halfway and try jumping to make a new list before you are through with the original. Sorry, but that will not work.

Whether you are reading this book on a screen or on paper does not make a difference. What is really important is that you do something to bring your worries on to a more material level. That's why it is important to make a concrete list, whether digitally or on paper. But not in your mind. You may well question that, and you may well be one of the fewer than 1% of the population who has a photographic memory; however for the vast majority of humans on this planet earth, it simply does not work to have this type of list simply in your mind. So, please write a list!

Once you have made a list you can then start planning how to reduce your daily dose of worry. Sounds strange? Perhaps, but just like you can start building your muscle power at any age, you can always start reducing your worry at any time. Spend time exploring your current high priority worry. Get to know it, get to know the colours, the smells, the sensations, the feelings of this worry. Inside and outside. Devote 15 minutes every day to this work, and then put it aside and go on with your daily life until tomorrow when you again look at your high priority worry. You may well be surprised one day to find that the particular worry is no longer a high priority. If so, then you can go on the next worry.

Fantastic pain! Who has not used that expression at some time or another? Of course it does not mean that the pain was simply a fantasy of my creative mind, it is usually used to describe a pain that came up during a particular action or situation that I feel good about describing to someone and often as a result of which I felt some kind of freedom, for example, the pain in my legs just before reaching the top of a steep hill which went away as soon as I cycled over the top!

Worry is something else. It does not simply go away if you try to ignore it. Worry tends to grow from lack of attention. It can also develop into anxiety and even go so far as to develop into various phobia which can even make it impossible to go outdoors. So, even if your worry is 'only' a product of your fantasy and exists only in your mind, that is no reason at all to ignore it! Worries are a bit like shadows, looked at from the corner of your eye during the twilight hours, shadows can sometimes look very dangerous. However, as soon as they are exposed to strong light, you laugh about the fantasy they brought up in your mind. Worries behave the same, look at them carefully, concentrate your attention on them, devote adequate time to really get to know them, and you will find that your worries will slowly get less and less dangerous and frightening and may even turn into friends; friends in the sense of acting as an 'early warning system' to give you advance notice that something needs to be looked at in your life.

Catherine was a worrier from childhood on but got concerned when she married and got her first child, Mark, and her worries started to take over her life as well as that of her son. So she decided to go into therapy and found a psychotherapist that she could talk to without anxiety. After some time Catherine was able to use her worries as a tool and one day was amazed to find that instead of worrying about her little boy dying from a cold, she was able to start taking care of her own health and had even started yoga classes and was delighted that Mark, her son enjoyed practising with her! She had learnt to use her life energy for the good of her family rather than waste it on worrying.

Some time ago the West European media was full of stories about 'multi-tasking', ranging from a woman on a bicycle on a high wire with a monkey on her head juggling with bananas to an old age pensioner who got into trouble with the police whilst reversing his car into his garage whilst using his mobile phone and ran over the neighbour's dog. The question is, how can you worry whilst doing your daily tasks? The answer is, don't even try! Worrying is such an important activity that it really deserves your undivided attention. Nothing more and nothing less.

This whole chapter has been devoted to the question of how to worry effectively, meaning basically how to get the most out of the time that you spend worrying. If that is really what you want, then, in a nutshell, the solution is...

Just do it.

Nothing else: just allocate a specific time each day to concentrate on your worries; they will reward you by reducing the consumption of your very own life energy, the energy that will then be set free for you to... To do what? Well, one of the ways you can use this energy that's been let loose, is to learn how to GLOW, and that is what the next chapter is about.

radiate

9 GLOW

About GLOW and glowing.

Glow. What is glow? Mostly it is defined as a source of light without a flame. Bear with me while I expand that notion. First, let's connect glow with the birth of light. In the beginning was glow, then came wind, the breath of life and through the breath/wind came the light of life.

Whether we accept this extrapolation or not, there does seem to be a universal acceptance that people who glow, or people who seem to have a glowing radiance about them, are desirable people to have around. Like charisma, it is indeed difficult to define but quite easy to experience. Both are of course subjective to a degree, but it is probably true that to be labelled a 'person who glows' or with 'a glowing personality' is a label that most people would like to have.

There is of course another aspect of glow. That is the inner feeling of glow. The feeling that we have when everything seems to function, to be 'right', when we are in tune with life. People who are not into touch, seldom glow. Really? Well that is my personal observation and it does not have very much to do with whether they are constantly touching others or being constantly touched by others. It has to do with being conscious or not that touching other human beings or being touched by other human beings is very, very important. There is a wonderful book on the subject by Ashley Montague, called 'Touching' where he goes very deeply into the subject. Look out for it.

We only have to look at the different attitudes towards human body contact in the eastern cultures of the world as opposed to the western. For instance, travelling by train in India you cannot help touching and being touched by others! If you sit alone on a long bench, the next person will sit right next to you. Whereas in Europe, people go to some lengths not to sit too close to you. There is of course a high level of neuroticism associated with human touch in western cultures, particularly in those cultures that practised physical beating of children as well as being very much against any form of sensuality and, of course, sexuality. It was only after the 'swinging sixties' and the liberalism of the 1970s that things started to change, at least in Europe, but there are still a lot of people around who are quite unhappy about being physically touched by others, whether as an expression of delight or simply as a greeting. Massage is still very much associated with antiquated concepts such as 'sin' or 'forbidden pleasure' in many western cultures, but fortunately that is slowly dying out.

Nuclear glow is very spectacular, but also very dangerous. Chernobyl and the explosion of the atomic power station there in 1986 served to remind millions of people in Europe that atomic energy can turn out to be a matter of life and death. 12 March 2011. In Fukushima, Japan the nuclear power plant exploded after the earthquake and the tsunami with the result that the anti-atomic power movement gained new impetus. One of the repair workers in Fukushima described how one of the most frightening aspects of the danger was that you could not see it. The explosion left marks, but the radiation danger was frightening simply because you could not see it, could not smell, taste or even feel it.

Maybe this secret and dangerous, but unknown, aspect played a role in Germany in the 1930s as Hitler and the Nazi party slowly built up a powerful organisation that at least on the outside, fairly glowed with hope and optimism for the future and blinded most of the populace to the dangers that lurked under the surface, until it was too late.

Isn't it strange that both sunburn and ice-burn feel the same? They both have a glow about them, just like the glow that comes after a cold shower. The big difference is that the glow that comes after a cold shower is pleasant whereas the glow after both sun- and ice-burn is often extremely painful.

On the other hand, the usual meaning of the term 'glow' is positive. If we look in the Oxford English Dictionary we find the following...

verb [no object]

give out steady light without flame: the tips of their cigarettes glowed in the dark; have an intense colour and a slight shine: [with complement]: a fluorescent screen glowed a faint green colour (of a person's face), appear pink or red as a result of warmth, health, embarrassment, etc.: he was glowing with health, convey deep pleasure through one's expression or bearing: Katy always glowed when he praised her.

noun [in singular]

a steady radiance of light or heat: the setting sun cast a deep red glow over the city. a feeling of warmth in the face or body: he could feel the brandy filling him with a warm glow. a redness of the cheeks. a strong feeling of pleasure or well-being: with a glow of pride, Mildred walked away.

Let's have a look at the above 'feeling of warmth in the face or body'. Many teenagers feel just that when they touch or are touched by a person they feel attracted to. Sometimes the warm glow is even too much, they get nervous or even afraid when the glow starts to turn on a sexual arousal process in their bodies. This can then turn into a challenging aspect of the relationship, particularly for those young people who grow up in a strict religious community where anything remotely sexual is seen as sinful. This is the point where the glowing experience can easily turn into a neurotic experience leading to later difficulties regarding issues of nearness in intimate relationships. What to do? It all boils down to one word, information. The younger one is when one is really informed about bodily processes, particularly sexual processes, the easier it is to deal with relationships involving intimate physical nearness. Of course it is never too late to learn, it's just that it usually takes longer to learn the older one is!

One of the problems of late learning is that there are so many tension spots in the body that have developed over the years that it is sometimes very difficult to learn to relax and, since a certain degree of relaxation is of utmost importance in an intimate relationship, this can possibly lead to numerous conflicts. The problem of unconscious tension in the physical body is something that Wilhelm Reich, a psychoanalyst and a student of Sigmund Freud, devoted many years into researching.

Have you ever experienced glow in your dreams? Carl Jung wrote a lot about archetypes in the collective unconsciousness and their manifestations in dreams. One example would be a holy person with a halo, that is a glowing circle of light around their head, similar to the glow of light that one can see during a solar eclipse. We could of course go on to explore the role of power in holiness and associate further with the image of the sun as a source of power, whether earthly or heavenly. In any case, the image of glow or glowing is something that often appears in the realm of fantasy and imagination. It seems to have a magical power to fascinate people through the ages and people keep on getting excited by glow from the early Egyptians right up to modern day religious processions where gold is often used to portray the glowing power of the deity. The reflected glow of sunshine from a gold-plated dome of a religious building has a power that can be seen from many kilometres away and the distance involved has a powerful influence on the people seeing it. Russia has many churches with golden domes. Very often they are of real gold leaf. It draws people to it. Something similar happens with human persons who have a glow around them, whether visible or not.

Is glowing of importance amongst friends? I really don't know about that but I do know that time is very important. In fact, time is the only thing that friends can give each other. The Scots and Quaker philosopher, John MacMurray, wrote a short essay about friendship pointing that out.

Time is also related to glow, in the sense that glowing is a phenomenon that often occurs spontaneously with certain babies and unconsciously by some very old persons. But on the whole, a person who emanates a glow around her has had to work quite a lot to establish it. The work that is necessary for the process of glowing to start is very much of an internal nature. It has little to do with cosmetic surgery and a lot to do with work on one's self. That takes time. We have established that normally the words 'glow' and 'glowing' have a mainly positive feel about them. On the other hand, we have seen that there are various examples of the words being used to describe situations and experiences that are not in themselves particularly pleasant. For example, being burned by a glowing piece of coal! Particularly when it comes to emotional feelings, I can think of many examples of persons really glowing with feelings of anger and hate towards others, particularly when it comes to questions of race and religion. In March 2011, during the uprisings in Libya, Colonel Gaddafi appeared on TV to be shaking with rage towards his fellow citizens who dared to disagree with him and fairly glowed with indignation that they did not believe in him any more. Does that mean that glow is bad? Not at all, it is just that we have to be somewhat careful when confronted with a clever, rhetorically experienced person with charisma so that we are not blinded by her glow and ignore the message that she is trying to impress on us.

When we have a fever, the body itself starts to glow. It gets hotter and hotter and feels more and more uncomfortable. Sometimes when near a person with a lot of spare energy, their simple presence sometimes seems to rob one of air, giving rise to a feeling of suffocating, a feeling which reduces radically when we create some physical distance between us and the person. In contrast to situations where the body starts to glow from inside, there are also circumstances like a storm where the action of cold wind and rain or sleet pounding the face can soon give rise to a feeling of facial glow, particularly when one stops in a sheltered place! Summer on the beach, lying in the warmth of the sun can also bring forth a very pleasant glow to the body.

Reading what I have just written, it seems, at first, rather banal but it is simply a further manifestation of the breadth of circumstances where glow plays a role in our every day life. Sometimes the inner glow is very small and one needs to blow on it to get it going. Sometimes one needs to keep on blowing on this tiny little glow for years, until it is strong enough to keep on going alone.

An interesting symbolical example is that of a blacksmith. His fire is based on coke, coal that has been pre-burned. The coke glows until the blacksmith or his helper starts working the bellows and then the glow becomes a very hot source that makes iron and steel malleable and being able to be formed into everything from scythes to swords. But it all started with a small glow.

Is there a special glow to do with women? Baroque churches are full of glowing madonnas; lots of gold and halos, in the sense of a circle of light behind or above a head of a person pictured in a painting or mural. Interestingly enough the word halo comes from the Greek, meaning disk, usually referring to the sun or moon. Even though the English word is very much associated with saints and holy people, the ancient Egyptians used the symbol to denote divinity or prestige of gods and rulers, so here we have various examples of relationships between light, sun, moon (light reflected from the sun), spirituality, holiness, divinity and persons. There is a glow that seems to be outside the person, much like that represented by the halo and that brings up the question of where it comes from. There was a period in time where people thought that a brilliant writer, artist or sculptor was a genius as opposed to a person who had, through hard and consistent work, been able to connect with the genius, the muse, the goddess, the divine, the creator.

That brings us to the particular time that we are in at the moment, the now represented by the 21st Century with Web 2, Internet, IT, electronic and technological communication, etc. You, the reader, are hopefully involved right now in a creative process. No? Why not? What is it that is stopping you from being pro-active, stopping you from tapping in to your own personal creative process, your own book, your own new artwork, song, business project. What is stopping you? Check out whether you have been caught up in the false concept that genius, the creative muse, the secret of success or whatever, is something that is pre-ordained, in other words you either have it or you don't. At this point I would like you to stop for a moment, consider the whole concept of glow and see if you can befriend yourself with the idea that you have a little seed buried inside you and you simply have to open yourself, to let the light come in, to touch the seed and let it grow. Could it be that the secret of glowing has to do with the interaction between you and your environment?

Having looked at glow in connection with the feminine whether in the form of the divine muse or in terms of the internalised archetype of the female, let's now look at men and glow. The most significant factors seem to be power, health and attraction. The Chinese culture has a neat way of symbolising the male /female dichotomy with yin and yang. But coming back to western concepts, men are still attracted to businesses like nuclear power stations, in spite of huge catastrophes like Three Mile Island, Chernobyl and Fukushima. It's rare indeed to find women in positions of power in this industry. Does the glow of a nuclear reaction appeal more to the male? Is it simply a question of education and society or has it got something to do with more fundamental issues? Do we have to consider male glow and female glow as two different aspects of one concept?

There is of course the question of androgynous glow. A prime example is David Bowie in the early years. He certainly glowed, but it was difficult to classify his glow as male or female, whereas someone like Mohammed Ali was, or still is, a predominantly male with a particular male glow about him.

The basic question is 'to glow or not to glow'?

Children on the other hand do not have to work particularly hard to be able to glow. Many, particularly small children seem to have a built-in natural glow about them but my observation is that they very soon undergo a process of socialisation that chips away at the glow until there's nothing left. There are many references in the New Testament about the importance of being like little children in order to glimpse heaven. Could be that it refers to innocence and trust, qualities that small children don't have to learn. One particular aspect of glow is that concerning glow and sickness. Some kinds of illnesses seem to engender a form of glow particularly around children. In Victorian times there was for instance a romantic association around children and young women suffering from tuberculosis, they were often described as glowing with passion.

Wyddost ti pwy wyt pan wyt yn cysgu?

Ai corff ai enaid, ai argell gannwyll?

Do you know who you are when you are asleep?

A body, a soul?

Or even a secret source of light?

This is part of a poem written by a mediaeval Welsh poet.

It raises the interesting question of the role of dreams in our soul or spiritual life, as well as the connection between life and light. Now we are back to the ancient Egyptians and their concept of the sun being the primary godhead. So is it any wonder that we associate a glowing personality with star-allure, that most of us are attracted to a person who has a certain glow about them?

During the course of this book we will be looking at ways of making you so open that you're inner glow will seek its own way out to appear on the surface of your being where, for those who are searching for it, it will be visible.

balance

10 WORK & GLOW

A look at applying glow principles at work.

Who was Dale Carnegie?

Dale Carnegie was a role model and teacher for at least two generations of males from the English speaking cultural world, and even though the man himself is long gone, his work, particularly in the realm of public speaking still lives on in various parts of the world.

He was also the author of a very successful book entitled 'How to stop worrying and start living'. It's a bit dated nowadays but was very influential in the 1940s and fitted well into the popular literature of the time.

One of the things that Dale Carnegie wrote about that is still relevant is the importance of listening to the other person. Don't you also find that it is a rare experience to meet someone who really listens to you? I recently watched a TV programme about Cassius Clay or rather Mohammed Ali as he is named now. One of the most endearing traits about this amazing person, who is still known and respected all over the world is that most of the people who have met him are very impressed that he listened to them and gave them the feeling that they were important.

Why not try listening, really listening to the next person you talk to? You might be surprised at what they have to tell you if you really take the time to listen!

The other important subject that Carnegie dealt with was self-confidence, and his particular method of dealing with it through public speaking. I was particularly fortunate in this respect in having a chemistry teacher who insisted on all his pupils learning to speak spontaneously for 5 minutes on all kinds of simple topics such as 'common salt' – a truly invaluable experience and one of the few remaining pleasant memories of my school days!

Even though Dale Carnegie is long dead, some of his basic concepts are still very relevant to life in the 21st century. The TED conferences are extremely successful and are based primarily on good quality public speaking!

One interesting aspect about the most attractive lectures is that the speakers are very interested in their topic and are lovingly enthusiastic when they talk about their favourite subject.

The academic scholars will describe this enthusiasm as a direct link to something of a godly (small case!) nature (from the Greek 'theus') which has the delightful side effect of making the speaker glow.

Enthusiasm is always extremely important when it comes to glowing. It is however important to differentiate between genuine enthusiasm arising out of pure interest in the subject on the one hand and the hollow interest pretended by others.

A particularly appealing example of an enthusiastic speaker and writer is Seth Godin, author of some really great books like 'Tribes' and 'The Purple Cow' and an impressive expert on life in the post-industrial Age of the Web. I particularly love getting his news mails through sethgodin.com. Some of them are highly informative, some amusing but all stand out because of the level of care that goes into them. I'm sure you know what I'm talking about when I refer to the gutter level of most so-called information mails!

Seth's mails often glow with the intensity of his commitment to the subject, somewhat similar to the glow emanating from a good carpet, picture or sculpture. It's the difference between living and not living.

There is a little phrase called 'positive thinking' that keeps on cropping up from time to time. I remember that there was a very successful speaker called Norman Vincent Peale who was around about the same time as Billy Graham the evangelist preacher, in the 1960s. There was also a Frenchman called Emile Coue who established in the early 1900s a psychological self help system based on autosuggestion and will power.

Interestingly enough, Coue seemed to have been amongst the first to look at the phenomena of the placebo effect. Coue's method was based on daily repeating a mantra:

Every day, in every way, I'm getting better and better.

It seems as if Peale and other modern American writers based their work very much on Coue's theories, which brings me to the following observation. Europeans are very creative when it comes to dreaming up new ideas from psychoanalysis to the atomic bomb or space rockets but it often takes Americans to transform the ideas into every day reality for the mass of people. An example of democracy in action?

I grew up in Wales where each and every family has family members who at some time or another emigrated to the USA, Canada, Australia or other parts of the old British Empire or colonies. For us then, the American cousins epitomised everything that was new and modern! Today I tend to think that the future can benefit from the creativity of people from all over the world combining with the technological design represented by companies like Apple to produce things like the iPad, which I am using to write this book on!

A great example of a new development in terms of the present positive thinking book market is Today We are Rich by Tim Sanders. Well worth reading. Available, of course as an e-book on Kindle!

Which brings us to the Internet, and the question of what has concepts like worrying or glowing to do with the world wide web?

At first glance nothing. However looking a bit deeper we find that many people use the web for communicating, for selling or just to gather information. Amongst the factors that play a role in the decision making process, in deciding which website to look at, the question of who glows more, or at least which person gives the impression of glowing more, seems to play a significant role. This is particularly true when it comes to video on the web.

Glowing is a very nice feeling to experience... just like what happened to me yesterday. I attended a public lecture at the university in Freiburg, in the Black Forest region of Germany, where Dr. Eckhard Rudiger spoke about the clinical methods of Schematherapy and presented his latest book on the subject. Having got an e-mail announcing the lecture the previous day I was curious to hear what he had to say, because he was one of the first patients in my new practice in Germany in 1981. Speaking to him afterwards, I was overjoyed to hear him bubbling over with joy at seeing me after all these years, and particularly as he went on to say that the therapeutic work with me in those early years just as he was starting on his medical career was of significant importance in defining his later work in the development of Schematherapy in Germany. He showed me his latest book 'The Practice of Schematherapy' and the dedication to me as the one who made sure that the author did not turn out to be quite such a bad father as his own. (in German – "Praxis der Schematherapie")

Well, you can imagine that on the way home I was fairly glowing, with pride, with affection, with recognition and with the particularly warm and glowing feeling that my work does sometimes have a long lasting effect. One of the paradoxes of modern mobility is that a psychotherapist working in a large metropolis rarely has the opportunity of hearing about the long term success of his or her individual work, the patients who return indicate only a short term success, the ones who do not return may well have gone somewhere else! They may well be at peace with themselves and with the world. It is however a rare occasion when they communicate this, unasked, to the therapist they saw many years ago.

But, you may well ask, does not the rapid growth of social networking, both within and without the Internet, open up endless possibilities to glow and get known and recognised within this truly world wide web of pop and alternative as well as, to an increasing extent, mainstream culture?

The Germans have a great expression: Jain! It means 'yes and no'. It applies very much to this question. The Web does mean that you can be in touch with many persons without having to be concerned about geographic restrictions. It does also mean that something is constantly and intrinsically missing from these relationships, the physical, bodily, living aspect of TOUCH.

Now touch is a very underrated factor in much of today's predominantly Western influenced culture. Even to the extent that, in 2011, if you were admitted to hospital in Germany, the chances are that, unless you needed surgery, no doctor would touch your body anywhere with his hands! You don't believe it! Well it is unfortunately true. In fact, very few medical students learn today how to touch their patients. A few do in fact rebel against this trend and start to learn how to touch patients even to the extent of experimenting with laying on of hands in cases where they find they are not getting further with their high-tech medicine.

I myself learnt this the hard way as, after closing my private practice in the city of Frankfurt in Germany, in 2006 I started a virtual practice using web-based video and audio technology and had to admit that it only worked well with persons with whom, at some point or another in time, I had a real, person to person, physical contact. Or had close contact with a common acquaintance. Looking back it is of course easier to explain, possibly in terms of bonding, but it took quite a long time before I even questioned the difficulties that I experienced in getting the virtual practice really up and running.

Work is, ideally, a life-long learning process. It was Piaget, I believe, who said that you can only learn if you make mistakes!

It has taken me an awful long time to grasp this simple truth. For instance, I often lectured in the 1970s about the importance of conscious direct physical contact between psychotherapists and their clients, whether or not it was limited to a handshake, a bear hug or intensive body work. However by 2006, I seemed to have completely forgotten this basic rule, which led of course to a series of very expensive business and economic mistakes.

Which brings me to the interesting topic of cyclic phenomena in the particular sense of, is it really necessary to touch rock bottom before you start reversing that direction?

Certainly in terms of health issues I tend to believe that people who experience serious illness as a child tend to be more aware of the importance of health in later years as compared to those who have always been healthy until one day they become ill in middle age or even later. Many end up being devastated by the new experience of being helpless in the face of pain and suffering.

One of the paradoxes of being quite ill as a child around the middle of the twentieth century in Britain was that I learnt a lot about time. Time? Yes, I was forced by circumstances to be alone most of the time when sick and had thus many opportunities to learn about the nature and the usage of time. Experiences that later proved useful in adult life as I began to explore subjects like contemplation and meditation.

Time is also extremely important in analytically oriented psychotherapy, when it is often necessary to go back in time to particular emotional experiences.

Sure, time heals lots of wounds and pains but sometimes it happens that time builds an armour over the memory of the experience, resulting, in the worst possible case, in the emotional feelings festering in the same way that a sick root of a tooth sometimes festers in the gum whilst the surface seems ok. The festering emotions can then lead to various psychosomatic disorders. A particularly dramatic form of this kind of disorder was treated by a Brazilian friend and colleague of mine, Lazlo Avila. The full account is available in the Proceedings of the 2009 Congress of the Groddeck Society of Germany, but it was basically about how a worrying experience can fester underneath the surface of a man's life and consciousness and result in a wound not being able to heal until the whole sad story of his youth was told to an understanding and sympathetic person, in this case, the person of the analyst Dr Lazlo Avila.

The extreme example noted above is relevant to the topic of work and glowing not only as a warning that not enough conscious attention can well lead to disastrous consequences, but also that conscious attention to a problem can often lead to a successful resolution. After one has successfully resolved a particularly difficult problem it can well be of value to extend one's spheres of interest into the community. The danger of ignoring the interests of the community (in whatever form it is defined) was illustrated by the case of Rupert Murdoch, the media tycoon, in 2011 when various executives of his media empire, News Corp., News of the World, etc. were forced to resign when it came out that some of their journalists spied, not only on celebrities of one form or another, but also on ordinary people, the kind of people who represent their paying customers. That was just too much for the community of customers, readers and media consumers. They stood up and shouted NO.

How can one serve the community in a helpful and positive way, appropriate to the 21st Century? It's impossible to define a universal recipe for this kind of service but a good starting point is your own back yard. By that I mean, try looking around your own local community for specific needs, whether material needs like food or shelter, emotional needs like loneliness, or even spiritual needs. Then do some research into what other people are doing to combat these or other needs. An appropriate next step could well be to approach these other active people which a view to joining them or to cooperate with them. If you are too shy or anxious to get involved locally then try looking on the Internet for ways to apply your own particular interests and skills in an appropriate way.

Giving to your own tribe/community, whether real or virtual, is a good first step to establishing your own glow. You may have heard of the saying that a lighted candle is one of the best gifts for a woman caught in the dark!

I remember years ago seeing newspaper ads saying 'be a man, expand your chest'. Now it may well be appropriate to say: be a woman, expand your interests.

This way you will certainly bring some glow into the life of your local community and you may well get some kick-back glow for yourself in the process.

Will charity work help me glow?

Charity and activism are two realms that often result in bringing some glow into the lives of people. Did you notice that I have slowly moved over into talking about generating glow for others rather than generating your own glow?

It is my experience that there are two basic processes involved.

A centripetal process where you as an individual concentrate on consciously improving your personal health through nutrition, exercises, spiritual and meditative disciplines and so on. This will prepare the ground for developing your inner glow, which may in the course of time emanate from your innermost being and be perceived as such by those around you. Somewhat in the sense of 'Gosh, look at her glowing with health on the pitch'.

Then there is a centrifugal process where you are responsible for bringing glow into the lives of others and through your efforts, the glow that develops in them radiates out and reflects from you.

Both these processes are valid and who is to say that one person or process is better than the other? It really does seem to me that any process or human being that contributes to increasing the amount of true glowing in the world is worthy of praise. We each of us do not have to go far away from home to discover someone who is more needy than us, someone who will surely appreciate and benefit from some thing that we have more than enough of. Please think about that.

How important is being self employed when it comes to glowing?

Service means different things to different people. In Germany a civil servant is called a 'Beamte' and is specifically there to serve the state. That leads to a lot of jokes about them being too tired to work! Behind these jokes is often a feeling that these are people who have given up on taking responsibility for their doing and are content to wait to be told what to do, in exchange for a secure pension when they grow old. This choice affects all those of us who work, whether or not we have an independent private income. One crucial factor is whether to be self-employed or not.

Certainly there are many activities that do not easily fall into this category. However, the basic question has to do with how do I personally feel about taking responsibility for what I do. Being self-employed is simply about taking 100% responsibility for what you do, with things like total freedom of choice in deciding your daily work programme, your long-term goals as well as your free time.

In practice that means that some people succeed in organising their life and work, doing what they really enjoy doing, with the result that they often glow and radiate a feeling of being at ease with their work and life; whereas others constantly suffer from stress trying to keep up with their work schedule and particularly with attaining their economic goals. This latter category often suffers because their whole business existence is based on material success whereas the first category mostly decide for self-employment as a means for realising their wish for working in a field that gives them a certain amount of satisfaction for their soul or spiritual existence.

Does an old boy/girl network help one to glow?

Networking plays a pivotal role in building a new business independent of whether you are working for spiritual satisfaction or primarily for material success. In the old, pre-millennium days, the 'old-boy' principle played a major role, being based on a circle of acquaintances and friends from school and college days who often proved useful in introducing one to people who could help establishing a circle of customers, clients, patients or whatever.

The twenty first century brought in a new, web based concept of social networking represented by Facebook and friends. One result is the growth of new means of marketing represented by such gurus as Seth Godin and his concept of building tribes of people with common interests.

2011 demonstrated for the first time the global impact of such organisation forms as they were significantly responsible for the peaceful demonstrations and the partly peaceful revolutions in the Arab World such as in Egypt, Tunisia etc. There is of course another side to this development and that is that these networks can also be used to propagate non-democratic, racist or other goals not in accordance with human rights principles.

On the other hand such networking can also be important in bringing together different cultures and nations with the one negative side effect that all have to use English as the basic language tool. However, based on the European experience, it can often lead to national sub-networks with an increasingly valuable contribution to the national culture without the danger of losing contact to the European or world communities.

Glow can sometimes be compared to the fable of the emperor's new clothes where only one little boy refused to believe that the king had invisible clothes on when he saw him walking through the streets with no clothes on. The little boy just saw a naked man walking and the others were so caught up in their own fantasy world that they only saw a magnificently clad emperor walking the streets!

Many so called celebrities have been imbued with an artificial aura that surrounds their media presence and which suddenly disappears when they appear before people who are not aware of their status.

Then there are the people with an inner glow in whose presence some others feel particularly comfortable without having a rational explanation for it.

Can one learn how to glow? Now that is a very interesting

question and I personally have come to the conclusion that the most one can do is to work on one's own individual infrastructure to ensure a fertile ground for personal growth. Then comes a certain amount of self-discipline and self-responsibility combined with a plan of action suited to one's own strengths and weaknesses. Then, whether you apply your talents to fashion, yoga, building bridges, playing rugby, surgical operations on human hearts, painting, writing or composing pop songs the important factor is that you are personally 100% involved in what you are doing. That means being consciously aware all the time of what you are doing.

This book attempts to give an overview of various approaches towards encouraging as well as fertilising your personal ground structure so that any germinal ideas that fall your way will not be automatically dismissed as useless.

According to my friend A, religious belief and faith seems to be a necessary foundation for a life assertive glowing feeling. He himself is a great example of a man who, in whatever company he finds himself in, whether a meeting of heads of state or a beach barbecue, emanates a glow of acceptance to those around him, resulting in him being greeted with friendly words and actions irrespective of his perceived or real influence or usefulness for the greeter.

During the course of a relaxed supper party one of his friends suggested that one of the main factors in the charm that makes A universally loved and respected is his conscious ability to switch from being a playful little boy larking around, to the serious and well informed, negotiator and mediator. Whatever the occasion, he is fully and consciously there, in the appropriate role.

Whether your life is based on faith or on humanistic

principles, it does seem to be quite important to try and live in the moment, with respect for the rights of other human beings to share the earthly space where you find yourself. That's the being part. As regards the doing part, it seems necessary to be concentrated and involved in your daily activity, whatever that is. One can usually recognise these people because they are so enthusiastic about their work and the material and financial element recedes into the background. Two quite simple rules, but not necessarily easy to practice, summed up as being and doing in the here and now.

Starting on the path to this goal is no guarantee that you will end up a glowing pillar in your community, but it will certainly be of help, even in just establishing a foundation for your efforts.

Will glowing help your career? Social networking is seen as the guarantee for business success in the twenty first century. However a bit of a glow in your personality will certainly not fail to be of value in gaining friends and influencing people on the way up the career ladder.

There are lots of business coaches out there, each with her own brand of techniques and methods designed to manipulate associates and colleagues as well as present or future bosses so that they perceive you in the best possible light.

However, all these methods demand a 100% commitment to the pre-determined material and financial goals and hardly any pay attention to your spiritual and emotional needs and interests. Consequently, there is a built in danger that you become successful but also dissatisfied, if your inner needs are not taken sufficiently into account.

As Susan, a client of mine once said, 'I'm sick and tired of talk, talk, talk all day long with only tiredness to show for it... talk about doing things for me that ends up mostly in talking and no doing'.

I think it was Seth Godin who once said that there is no
such thing as a conscientious company, only individuals
can have a conscience, not a firm! We still have not created an emotional feeling computer, even though my darling
iPad does come a bit closer to it! If we think of paradise
or heaven as concepts that have to do with peace of mind,
then it is not surprising when the Bible talks about a busi-
nessman having an easier time getting through a small
opening the size of a needle head as opposed to getting
to heaven. It must surely refer to those whose only goal
in life is getting more and more money, no matter what it
costs in human terms. Someone even suggested that the
Bible really condemns the greed for money rather than
money itself. In other words, greed for money is the root
of all evil as opposed to money being the root of all evil.
That's really something to think about, isn't it?

Glow that truly comes from inside is something that you
perceive whether the person is rich or poor. In the world
of glowing the state of your bank account has no relevance.

Is there insurance for loss of glow in old age? Very old
people, or rather, some very old people radiate an inner
glow of their own. My grandmother was over 90 years of
age, in bed on doctor's orders, recovering after being taken
ill with influenza or something like that and I, a teenager then, was visiting her. She was lying in bed between
snow white sheets and radiated such light that I was very
perplexed at the phenomena. Her parchment-like skin
seemed to be illuminated from within and glowed with a
white intensity. She told me that she felt superfluous and
saw no point in living if it just meant lying in bed all the
time. This from a woman who was never seriously ill, was
widowed young in life, never re-married and managed a

sizeable detached house on her own until a couple of years previously, when she was more or less forcibly removed into the care of her daughter, my aunt. What was it? I do not know, except that she died soon after. Maybe the last surge of energy before the candle of life was extinguished? In any case a gripping and fascinating experience for me.

Here I am sitting in bed, enjoying the first morning rays of sun on the Black Sea coast of Bulgaria, having passed the mark of biblical life expectancy by a couple of years, writing about my grandmother and thinking that the prospect of facing death has lost its aura of fear for me and wondering at the relevance of such remarks for a book about worry and glowing!

Before we start going further into the question of possible fear of death maybe we should look a bit more closely at the question of the fear of life. Fear of life? Yes indeed, most people are quite afraid of living their life to the full. Afraid of being brave. Afraid of taking risks. Afraid of burning their boats, bridges or even breeches. Most people are quite simply afraid of living their life to the full.

Is there a connection between glow and spiritual work? Religious art, or at least traditional religious art is full of haloes around the heads of saintly and holy figures, even as far back as the Egyptians. Which brings up the question of whether there is a connection between the sun and the conception of holiness. Just look at a picture of the sun in eclipse and you will see a pulsating glow emanating from the surface of the sun. Superimpose a painting of a human head on top of the sun and you get a picture of a saintly person.

That's probably enough about working and glowing for now, so let's look at glow and time in the next chapter.

stop

11 WHEN TO GLOW?

Time and the Age of Glowing

"There is no time but the present."

"Here and now."

"Live for the moment."

"Only those who are like children have a chance of going to heaven."

What have all these phrases in common? They all refer to a phenomena that such varied persons as Gautama Buddha, Jesus Christ, George Fox, Carl G. Jung, amongst others, have spoken about. It has to do with a very simple but very difficult and challenging task. A task which small children have no difficulty with. Living in the exact time that you find yourself in. Not thinking or feeling about the past. Not thinking or feeling about the future. Just being fully, with mind, body and soul, in the present moment. Tell a small child that it will get an ice cream tomorrow and for her that means an eternity, meaning never. We as adults, on the other hand, are mostly either dwelling on our past actions or wishing about our future, but rarely are we in the present. Time. Have you ever thought about time? About what it means to you personally? What do you associate with the word time? Spend a minute or two of your time thinking about your own particular, personal views, thoughts, feelings relating to that word, that very simple word, time. Maybe you realised the intimate connection with memory. Which reminds me of a story an old friend of mine, called Bruno Martin, told me years ago.

Bruno was a one time student of a pupil of Gurdjieff and was given the following mental exercise. Spend the whole day NOT thinking about pink elephants!

Isn't it a marvellous exercise?

As you have probably realised by now, even though it sounds quite simple to say 'I will live in the here and now', in practice it is not so easy. The 'how to' part of it is something that a lot of people have worked on over the centuries. From the early Druids who pointed out the difficulty of finding the exact point at which the mistletoe plant changes into the host tree, to the early Egyptians who were very aware of time and the importance of timing. From Jesus Christ with his metaphor of children and heaven, knowing that small children live very much in the present before their consciousness has fully realised the concept of time, of past and future; to C.G. Jung who wrote copiously about the importance of living in the here and now. One of the most effective ways of consciously experiencing and developing the state of mind of being fully in the present is through the practice of meditation, specifically through the practice of Vipassana meditation, the art of meditation developed by the Buddha and transmitted over the centuries through various monasteries and schools, primarily in Myanmar, Sri Lanka and parts of India.

How can you glow in the morning? Well, let's start with looking at how to be in the morning. Or rather, how to be right now.

STOP

Yes, stop whatever you are doing right now and feel your body. Feel that part of your body that touches something or someone else. What is under your feet? What is under your buttocks? What are you in touch with? Listen! What do you hear? Listen again; what is in the distance; what's near by? Smell! Yes, just smell what's near your nose, what's around you, what's further away? Close your eyes. What do you see in your imagination?

Do you get the idea?

Do you notice that it really is possible, even for a short period of time, to be fully in the present as long as you are able to fully concentrate on the task at hand.

You might like trying to develop a morning ritual based on spending a period of time, long or short, practising being fully focussed on one particular sensory experience, whether the sense of touch, of smell, of taste, of...

If you ever find yourself experiencing sunrise you might be astonished at how the glow of the morning sun gradually grows to fill the sky. Later on we shall be looking at how this glow has fascinated people through the centuries, even to the extent of picturing persons deemed to be holy with the image of the glow of the sun behind their heads, the halo of religious art.

Japan, the land of the rising sun has incorporated this phenomenon into its entire culture and philosophy.

Who glows in the afternoon? The British Empire at the height of it's glory, or power, depending on your perspective, advertised itself as the realm where the sun never sets. It even glowed with pride and pleasure at the holy ritual of tea-time. But, joking apart, it does seem that a certain amount of ritual or ritualised behaviour can be useful in terms of preparing you for the kind of inner strength that seems to play a role in the life of persons who glow.

Habitual repeating of a certain kind of behaviour, whether it's cleaning your teeth after getting up or storing your car keys in a particular place, can be useful because it introduces an element of automation into actions that are basically dull but useful. It also can lead to a more effective use of time and energy. People who are always hectic and tense, never glow with a sense of inner peace; they are often those who are constantly looking for lost keys or are always late for important appointments but with long complicated explanations or excuses.

If we assume that the efficient use of our available life energy is a worthwhile goal, then you might like to spend some time considering ritualising some things in your life. If you are writing a book, most authors are agreed that it is important to spend a certain amount of time every single day on writing. Not preparing or researching, just on writing. In that case you might like to make a ritual based on a specific time to start and to stop, for instance.

Do spend some time thinking about your life goals and

then how you can ritualise some of the daily steps that are necessary for you to reach that goal or goals.

Do you look forward to evening time? Why? Is it because you can stop working for the day? So you can have a drink at your local bar, meet friends, go to an after-work party or something else? The evening is also a time when the glow worms come out, or at least the time when one can see them. They may well be around the rest of the day but there is something quite magical about seeing glow worms moving sedately around in that twilight zone before it gets really dark.

Evening is the time for networking, for making contact. It is the time when those who glow have a distinct advantage, whether it's in trying to get a drink at a crowded bar or a table at a busy restaurant. Imagine yourself being introduced to some people that you have been interested in. People that could be very valuable career or business contacts. Imagine what impression you are going to make on them if you have just emerged from a sweaty, aggressive meeting where your current dream project has been trampled down on, or if you have just had a good workout followed by a sauna. Which preparatory activity will help you glow? No prizes for the correct answer.

Night time is something else, it is traditionally the time for romance. A time where the glow of the setting sun, the glow of a candle or even the glow of hidden lights in a night club can arouse tender and romantic feelings and emotions in even the hardest souls. Have you ever wondered why that is? Why should a state of being centred around a physical phenomena that makes it difficult to differentiate between various silhouettes, even between different spaces, people and animals, be associated with romance?

Are we moving here in a direction away from the factual, the rational, the logical, into the world of the irrational, the illogical, into a dream world?

Is in fact, the whole concept of glow, of glowing simply a fantasy, a product of our imagination?

Maybe. But it is nevertheless a very real phenomena. However, the associative thoughts and concepts related to glow and glowing do certainly vary depending on the cultural concept. Recently a dear friend of mine complained about the constant state of twilight in many orthodox Christian churches and said that, for her, churches should always be full of light. This is where we come to the crux of the matter. Even though glow is a physical material phenomena, it is very much a question of individual subjective taste and opinion, as to it's meaning for you personally.

Try to think for a minute about what appealed to you in the title of this book, was it the prospect of reducing your worry or increasing your glowing?

Even though associated, they are not two sides of the same coin and reducing worrying is no guarantee that you will start to glow. The bridge between the two concepts has certainly to do with emotional feelings and that is certainly a theme that we shall be looking more closely at in this and other chapters.

Is it natural to glow as a child? There are some children who glow and some who do not. Certainly in religious art, particularly in Orthodox Christian iconic art, the Christ-child is always portrayed with a glowing halo around his head. In many cultures a glowing child symbolises the very essence of innocence and purity. Similarly the young green budding leaves in Spring give the forest a glow that is quite unique.

Whether it is a natural characteristic for children to glow is doubtful.

It does seem that if a small child is lovingly cared for, then it does have a very good chance of ending up glowing or at least with the potential for glowing.

Which brings us to the question of power and responsibility. By its very nature a small child is dependent. Dependent on someone to feed, wash and clothe it. Which in turn makes for ample opportunities for those in or with power to use that power to harness the energies of those children in their hands. The poor, the innocent, the weak have always suffered under unbridled power. On the other hand, the poor, the innocent, the weak have the power to glow in an atmosphere of loving care.

Did you ever notice that some teenagers are withdrawn, shy, seemingly always in a bad mood and unfriendly?

Some, on the other hand, resemble Aegia, the 'healthy glow', one of the daughters of Asclepius, the god of medicine and healing in ancient Greece religion. Having recently been to the Thalassic plain in central Greece where Asclepius reportedly lived, I can well imagine that some of the young people there, with their healthy glow, could easily have been mistaken for young gods and goddesses!

Nearby is also Mount Olympus and the original source of the Olympic Games, the prototype gathering of young, healthy, glowing athletes.

Coming back to Asclepius: The temples of healing in ancient Greece associated with the cult of Asclepius are also of interest because the patients spent the night in the holiest part of the temple and their dreams were interpreted by a priest to establish the appropriate form of therapy for the individual, a forerunner of psychoanalysis.

Even the original Hippocratic Oath started with Apollo and Asclepius swearing to practice in an ethical manner; so we can see that from ancient times there was a connection between glowing and being or becoming healthy.

Flow and glow seem to be related. If you ever have the opportunity to see the very original water fountain created in London's Hyde Park as a memorial to Lady Diana, Princess of Wales, you really can experience the connection between the water flowing, seemingly in two directions at the same time, and the extraordinary effect that she had on people all over the globe. In spite of, or because of her very humanness, she was able to flow through the minefields of the world as well as in high society ballrooms.

Another glowing person who mastered the art of flowing was David Lloyd-George, the Welshman who became the British Prime Minister during World War 1 and the man who was one of the first to address the need for health, education and social services for the poor and for the newly emerging class of industrial workers. He was able to flow between political power and his Welsh upbringing. It was his 'Welshness' that sensitised him to the immense cultural potential in the working classes, and was based on his experience of the glowing cultural life of the North Wales slate industry workers at the turn of the 19th and 20th centuries.

But there are also examples of really evil people who were or even are, capable of glowing. One example is Adolf Hitler whom countless observers described as having eyes that glowed with passion and that seemed to have a hypnotic effect on many. So maybe we have to be careful when using the term glowing in a purely positive sense. Perhaps we need to make sure of the context and the actions of the person who glows before we allow ourselves to be blinded by the glow that emanates from them! 'All that glitters is not gold' is an old proverb that seems to fit in this situation. However, we all know that it is not always easy to be objective when it comes to classifying a person as being good or bad. How often have we been disappointed, angry or sad on finding out something bad about a person whom we had always thought of as being intrinsically good.

One person that has a global reputation of being a good person is Jesus Christ. Even though not always recognised as being holy, he is nevertheless recognised as being good as opposed to evil. In Christian art he is often portrayed with a halo, a circular glow behind or above his head. This particular symbol is originally derived from the sun, the ultimate glowing disc constantly emanating energy, heat and light to give life to people on earth.

When you were a baby, the chances are that as long as you were born healthy, you started to emanate a glow like most newly born babies. However, as soon as the process of maturation, or growing up, starts, then a process of de-glowing begins. Just look around you amongst the adult people; are they glowing? Do they give off an aura of passion, awareness, focus? Or do they look bored, anxious, worried or tired?

Depression is often described as being a black state, a situation with no light at the end of the tunnel, not even a glow. That is the reason why someone who is depressed does not glow. There have been, over the years, various theories and practices addressing this problem. They range from Emil Coue, a Frenchman at the beginning of the 20th Century who suggested repeating a 'mantra' on the lines of 'every day little by little, I am getting more and more healthy'. William James, the famous American psychologist and philosopher, suggested, at about the same time, putting a smile on your face to start the day on the grounds that looking happy and glowing will slowly change your mental state from depressed to happy and glowing. There is no doubt that, provided your mental state can be defined as a 'temporary feeling of being downcast' as opposed to being clinically depressed, such techniques can be very valuable. The various methods loosely defined as 'positive thinking' owe a lot to Coue and James.

You may think that I am disparaging about these types of methods, but actually I find them OK but only as a sort of cosmetic treatment suitable for temporary emotional states that could be described as 'feeling a bit down', as opposed to clinical depression.

My paternal grandmother was not a very warm person, in fact she was emotionally frigid as far as I could make out. However she lived to the ripe old age of 93 without being really ill once. Just a few weeks before she died, I visited her when I was a young student and was astonished to find her in bed, emanating a sort of glow of white light. Quite extraordinary, particularly bearing in mind that I had normally only seen her dressed in various shades of black. Anyway, there she was, lying in bed and bathed in this light, telling me that she was not going to live long because 'they don't let me do a thing'!

What effect has our personal biographical history on the capacity to glow? Now that is a question that has been in my mind for a very long time and was recently satisfactorily resolved. It started in 1943 in a TB Sanatorium in the Denbigh Moors in North Wales. TB, tuberculosis, is a disease that was often used in novels in various cultures in the last half of the 19th century as well as the first half of the 20th century as a synonym for a romantic illness, full of images of sensitive young people living out their tragic destinies. It was quite well suited for the role because TB used to be characterised by a slow wasting away of life energy often accompanied by a perceived glow enveloping the whole person. For example, in Magic Mountain, a novel by Thomas Mann.

Now just imagine a small boy, just six years old, in exactly this situation! Add to that an image of a hospital built in the style of an Edwardian country house and estate, set in a park landscape and you have all the ingredients for a romantic, sensitive and tragic novel.

If you have read the introduction to this book, you will know what happened to this little boy in this Sanatorium.

Now jump forward 71 years, from 1943 to 2014 and accompany me on my journey into the past. I went by car to the village near Llangwyfan, on the Denbigh Moors, North Wales where the TB sanatorium was, a long time ago. The hospital was closed down in the 1970s, the buildings were empty for some time and then around about the late 1990s they were acquired by a private company and are now a clinic for mental health patients. Very nicely restored and renovated, it is an idyllic place surrounded by unspoilt nature.

It was with a feeling of relief that I realised that my particular memories of the peaceful effect the goldfish pond had on me are reflected by present reality. It was a secret place of recuperation, away from the illnesses, the misery and the deaths that surrounded me most of the time.

Another trip in the 'time machine' – this time to the late 1980s in Germany. I bought an old ruin of a house, a run down dilapidated one time hotel with a dream of opening a training centre for natural therapy and psychotherapy. The dream did not materialise but I did learn to re-connect with nature by working in the garden and landscaping the grounds. Sounds trivial doesn't it? But it wasn't.

It was a very significant experience and can be directly related to my finding solace as a six year old in that safe corner of nature in the park landscape of Llangwyfan.

Of particular significance is also the fact that re-visiting the site of my childhood trauma, the re-confirming that my memory of the beauty of nature there was correct, was important in confirming that the long-term suppressed memories of pain and hurt were also correct. This particular factor, one's own sceptic attitude to one's own experience of pain and hurt, is of importance in the therapy of people who suffered trauma in their childhood. The human organism is incapable of retaining memory of pain (actually a good thing if you think about it) and so it makes one vulnerable when it comes to sharing experiences from the past; one tends to retreat into one's shell when confronted with questioning disbelief.

That is why this trip into my past was useful for me in many ways. I am now of an age where you are more or less constantly confronted with the question of death and dying. This trip was another step in strengthening the spiritual foundation of my life, one of the building blocks being a quotation from George Fox, the Quaker: "there is no time but the present".

Both my parents are dead but in no way does that mean that they have ceased to exist for me. I sometimes find myself behaving like a headmaster telling off a naughty pupil, rather than asking the person why they did so and so. It does seem to me that my father certainly lives on as a part of me whether I want to or not. My mother, on the other hand, is still present as a separate entity that I sometimes find myself thinking it would be nice to telephone her, in order to share some experience or other.

So, what are you doing, yes, what are you doing, right now,

to make sure that you are living YOUR life?

Have you even thought about the possibility?

Just try asking yourself the very simple question: "What would my life look like if I was truly living my own life? What would I be doing right now, at this very moment? What would I look like? What would I be feeling?"

One thing is certain, the chances of you glowing with energy, with life energy, will be quite minimal if you do not even try to live your own life!

I can

12 THE GLOW TECHNIQUE

How to start glowing.

G L O W

G = go for it

L = love it

O = open your self

W = will your whole being

So, what does that mean in practice?

'**Go for it**'. Whatever you decide to do with your life, stay with it, go for it, go for this goal with all your strength, all your will, all your emotional energy. That is what 'go for it' means. It is that simple and that difficult!

'**Love it**' should be self-explanatory, but just in case it isn't, let's spell it out. It is no use being half- hearted when it comes to glowing. You really have to be in love with the idea. You have to be obsessed by the idea. You have to think of nothing else, at least for a while!

'**Open your self**'. Now that is somewhat more difficult to define and definitely more difficult to achieve.

'**Will your whole being**'. That means using everything, every single cell that you have.

Go for it:

Do you really think that you have understood the principle? You may well be right, but for the ones who are not so sure, a word of advice. Do not be afraid of making mistakes, do not be afraid of doing something wrong. That is the only sure and certain way to learn. Look at your mistakes, be aware of what exactly you did wrongly. Then you will have learnt something, you might even take a chance or two and make some bigger mistakes and you might end up learning even more. The one and only rule in this game is to keep on doing, to keep on exploring, to keep on learning. Playing safe and doing nothing will get you nowhere. Nowhere. Please remember that.

Love it:

In practice that means being prepared to devote both time and energy to the task of living your life to the full every second of the day. Impossible you might say. Yes indeed you may well be right. But that is no reason to stop trying. Have you ever been so engrossed in a particular activity that time just seems to fly? That is usually a sign that you are fully concentrated on what you are doing. That in turn is what we mean when we say that we love to do a particular activity. Now, if you really want to glow, you have to concentrate on everything and anything that you do, whether it's something like washing up, laying the table for one or choosing a new app for your smartphone.

Open your self:

I suppose it means being aware of what you are thinking, what you are feeling emotionally, being aware of what you are really experiencing in this world.

So much for my attempt at defining it. Sounds quite simple doesn't it? But, like so many things, difficult to achieve for any length of time.

Will your whole being:

Will your whole being. Now what the hell does that mean? Firstly it means that you have to use not only your head but your physical being, that means your body amongst other things, as well as your soul or psyche. It also means getting away from the goal of being holy. You remember that we noticed that the glow of a halo around the heads of wise or holy persons represents or seems to represent, an enlightened being? That is not the goal of the Glow Technique. The book and the technique is simply here to give you some clues about being more human, about being more of the person that you were born as, with the good as well as the bad parts, with your strengths as well as your weaknesses. However, it is important to be aware that you can do or be anything in the world that you personally can imagine, only as long as you believe that the following words are true as applied to you:

I can and I will

This book as well as the Glow Technique can certainly
be helpful when it comes to exploring the How, but the
only person who Can is going to be you and you can only
achieve that if you Will!

Some of the principles that form the base for glowing:

- Stop whatever you are thinking now.

- Breathe and be aware of it.

- Meditate a little but often, rather than a lot but rarely.

- Wait and listen to how life flows into you through the
  air that you breath.

- Listen to what is happening, in addition to the noise
  in your head.

- Digest what you have just experienced.

- Act, meaning be pro-active, just when the going gets
  tough, instead of being passive.

- Think about your favourite principles that fit into this
  scheme.

Before you can tune in to and hear your favourite radio or TV programme, you must turn the device ON. Some of us get so lazy that we don't search for a new programme but stay with the one that we have always tuned in to. Maybe its time to have a look at what else is going on; it might be interesting. Try listening to music you do not know, try being aware of what it does to you, of where it takes you, to the emotional feelings that are turned on by it. Practice being aware.

Feelings can bring you close to another state of consciousness, to another state of awareness, can bring you close to your soul, your spirit, maybe even to the godliness that lies hidden inside you. Did I hear you say 'Blasphemy'? Hang on a minute, I did not say that you are God, I simply referred to the godliness that you may discover inside you, not outside you. We are not referring to old concepts of old men living up in the sky, we are trying to look at the possibility of your discovering inside you something in addition to mathematical formulas, something other than abstract concepts developed for educating workers at the beginning of the industrial revolution. We refer here to the sacredness that lies at the very core of your particular self. OK you have difficulties with the word sacred or the concept of sacredness? Well, we are talking within the realm of religion or spiritual thought and belief systems. If that is really something you are allergic to then you are possibly reading the wrong book. Because even though I believe that all about and within me comes to an end when I die and even though I do not believe in concepts such as heaven or hell or transmigration of souls or reincarnation, I do believe in something of godliness that is hidden inside each and every human being on this earth, maybe in each and every sentient being. Whether we refer to that as religion or spirituality is not relevant. What is relevant is the idea that we are more than the sum of the material parts that we are constructed from. Personally I really like the word 'godliness' because, written in lower case, it leaves the meaning open to the individual interpretation with an infinitely large number of possible nuances, depending on the culture you were brought up in. Central to the concept that I am describing is the idea of self-responsibility with all its pro and cons as opposed to the idea of Gods and Goddesses ruling our lives. This particular sermon is now over.

Your body is the centre of your being. It is your factory, your studio, your workshop and your temple depending on whether you use it or not. Sure, we start off with different models, some in good shape and some not really suited to life on this earth as we find it when we take our first breath. But let's assume that you are more or less alive, that your body is more or less under your control and that you as an individual can more or less determine what you can do with or to your body in terms of feeding and exercise. What are you doing right now? Are you really reading these lines or are you jumping forward and thinking about what to do next, or are you worrying about what you have not done.

Turning on your mind means focussing on the task in hand, whether it is reading this book or climbing a dangerous rock face. With one small difference; not concentrating on climbing could lead to the loss of life or limb in a very clear way, whereas not concentrating on reading this or any other book only means an intangible loss. A potential loss, which is impossible to quantify because it depends very much on what you might have done with the information that you would have received if you had read it. Which reminds me of something John Cage wrote in his diary. He was writing about a Zen Buddhist teacher called Susuki who basically introduced Zen to America. Before Susuki started to meditate he saw mountains that looked like mountains. After many years and having reached a certain stage of consciousness he again saw mountains that looked like mountains. The difference was a change in perspective due to his being a fraction of a millimetre away from the earth!

In the same vein, C.G. Jung spent twenty odd years exploring his inner life and documenting his journey in 'The Red Book' which ultimately led to his particular form of psychological analysis called Analytical Psychology, as opposed to the psychoanalysis of Sigmund Freud. However, in all those years of self-exploration, Jung's relationship to his children was such that his children did not notice any significant change in their father.

When I was around fifteen years of age I discovered the joys of cycling. Up to that point, about the only two sports I was any good at were running short distances and table tennis. Cycling was a revelation for me; I could do it for as long as I wished, I did not have to look for a partner, and my parents gave me the necessary bicycle as a birthday present. Of course I did have a simple, fixed gear bicycle which was OK for my needs up to the time of revelation. But as soon as my eyes were opened I had to have a proper bicycle. In those days, the early 1950's in Britain, that meant a hand made frame from Claud Butler and a minimum of three gears from Campagnolo. Bicycling helped to turn on my body, made me fit and enabled me to enjoy the energy that flowed within me after a few hours cycling through the mountain passes of North Wales. This paradisiacal phase of my teenage years came to an abrupt end as I reached the age of eighteen and discovered the joy of motorcycling! But that is another story.

In the 1960s there were two main paths to turning on your soul. One was through drugs and the other by meditation.

I experimented with both and found meditation to be my tool of choice when it came to exploring my soul, and drugs when it came to exploring my senses. Meditation has stayed with me and drugs have stayed on the wayside for quite a few years now. Find your own tool, please.

This chapter opened with the suggestion of 'opening your self'. What on earth do I mean when I say to you 'open your self'? Try first of all looking into your thinking mind to see what words, feelings, pictures come up when you focus on the word 'open'. These are the things that you associate with open. That will give you a clue as to what opening your particular mind means to you personally. Really that's what it is all about. This book is not about people in general, it is about you in particular. It's a 'how to' manual that you have to programme to suit you personally. If you came up with words, feelings or pictures associated with the word 'open' these can be the starting point for you to explore the concept of opening your mind, of beginning to open your self. We can roughly divide them into three categories. Positive, negative, neutral. If they are positive you just need to carry on reading and you will certainly find other clues, which will help you in your quest. If, on the other hand, your associations were negative, by which I mean they were centred around unpleasant feelings or ideas, you probably need to spend a bit of time looking at your motivations for reading this book. Maybe you will find a conflict such as: 'I would love to learn how to stop worrying but am afraid to look too deep inside me just in case its horrible'. If that is the case, try reading the book slowly and look for passages which you find attractive, and then concentrate on these passages. I am not here to force you to 'face up to' your fears and anxieties! I am simply here, in the form of this book, to accompany you on your journey. You can, at any moment, decide how deep or how high or how broad or narrow you want to go. Try to remember the words of Gandhi: "The journey is the goal".

Let's now have a look at the idea of opening up your body. Let's start by feeling inside your mouth with your tongue. Did you ever realise that you actually have a tunnel inside you which goes from your mouth, via your throat, your stomach, your guts, your bowel directly to your anus. This tunnel, also known as the digestive tract, is where food is converted into energy and waste. There are also two other related types of 'tunnels', one of which works with drinking and liquids and one with breathing and air. According to traditional Chinese medicine, there are also channels or paths of energy called meridians. Depending on your interest and curiosity as well, of course, on your sense of adventure, you might like to experiment with looking at the effect of various food stuffs on your body. Fasting, either with fruits, juices or just plain water can sometimes be a particularly adventurous way of exploring your body and its relationship to your mind.

Opening up your soul is a way that traditionally has been associated in many cultures with fasting. Even though superficially, fasting seems to imply foregoing something, but that is only part of the picture. It also means getting rid of ballast, of unnecessary baggage. You only have to look around you to be aware that an increasing amount of human beings on this earth are carrying around with them every day a lot of excess baggage. Meditation, particularly the Vipassana tradition with its emphasis on observing the physical body, is a well-tested method of exploring the realm of soul and spirit.

Do you have a long past to look at? Even if you were born 25 years ago you still have a quarter of a century experience of living on this earth. Nowadays many authorities accept that the first five years of our life on this earth are extremely important in laying patterns of behaviour that influence our adult life. It is not a bad idea to look back at your early years from time to time and check up on possible influences that make life difficult for you in this day and age.

Try looking around you right now. Look out of the window if you are inside or just look around you if outside. What do you see? Close your eyes, try to conjure up what you have seen, then open your eyes and check the view. Look again, this time with some more attention and you may well find that you missed some things the first time.

Now listen around you. First with eyes open and secondly with your eyes closed. Notice a difference? You may well have heard something else with your eyes closed! It has to do with focussing your senses, in this case your sense of hearing, through shutting down your sense of seeing by closing your eyes. The phrase 'to be here and now' is often used to dramatise the need to aware of the present time. The need to focus on the present has always played a very important role in spiritual practices whether in being conscious of one's breath such as in various Eastern forms of mediation, or as described in the writings of C. G. Jung on the practice of analytical psychology and the need to constantly try to be here now even though in terms of practical every day life in the working places of the world today it is nearly impossible.

Many people have difficulty in staying in the present. We tend to either rummage around in our past or dream about a better future.

The problem with dreaming about the future is that the dream might just happen. Be very careful what you wish for. Don't know what I am talking about? Then spend a few of your precious minutes reading this fairy tale collected by the Brothers Grimm:

Once upon a time a woodcutter lived happily with his wife in a pretty little log cabin in the middle of a thick forest. Each morning he set off singing to work, and when he came home in the evening, a plate of hot steaming soup was always waiting for him.

One day, however, he had a surprise. He came upon a big fir tree with strange open holes on the trunk. It looked somehow different from the other trees, and just as he was about to chop it down, the alarmed face of an elf popped out of a hole.

"What's all this banging?" asked the elf. "You're not thinking of cutting down this tree, are you? It's my home. I live here!" The woodcutter dropped his axe in astonishment.

"Well, I.. ." he stammered.

"With all the other trees there are in this forest, you have to pick this one. Lucky I was in, or I would have found myself homeless."

Taken aback at these words, the woodcutter quickly recovered, for after all the elf was quite tiny, while he himself was a big hefty chap, and he boldly replied: "I'll cut down any tree I like, so..."

"All right! All right!" broke in the elf. "Shall we put it this way: if you don't cut down this tree, I grant you three wishes. Agreed?" The woodcutter scratched his head.

"Three wishes, you say? Yes, I agree." And he began to hack at another tree. As he worked and sweated at his task, the woodcutter kept thinking about the magic wishes.

"I'll see what my wife thinks..."

The woodcutter's wife was busily cleaning a pot outside the house when her husband arrived. Grabbing her round the waist, he twirled her in delight.

"Hooray! Hooray! Our luck is in!"

The woman could not understand why her husband was so pleased with himself and she shrugged herself free. Later, however, over a glass of fine wine at the table, the wood-cutter told his wife of his meeting with the elf, and she too began to picture the wonderful things that the elf's three wishes might give them. The woodcutter's wife took a first sip of wine from her husband's glass.

"Nice," she said, smacking her lips. "I wish I had a string of sausages to go with it, though..."

Instantly she bit her tongue, but too late. Out of the air appeared the sausages while the woodcutter stuttered with rage.

" What have you done! Sausages. What a stupid waste of a wish! You foolish woman. I wish they would stick up your nose!" No sooner said than done. For the sausages leapt up and stuck fast to the end of the woman's nose. This time, the woodcutter's wife flew into a rage.

"You idiot, what have you done? With all the things we could have wished for." The mortified woodcutter, who had just repeated his wife's own mistake, exclaimed: "I'd chop..." Luckily he stopped himself in time, realising with horror that he'd been on the point of having his tongue chopped off. As his wife complained and blamed him, the poor man burst out laughing.

"If only you knew how funny you look with those sausages on the end of your nose!" Now that really upset the wood-cutter's wife. She hadn't thought of her looks. She tried to tug away the sausages but they would not budge. She pulled *again and again, but in vain. The sausages were firmly attached to her nose. Terrified, she exclaimed: "They'll be there for the rest of my life!"*

Feeling sorry for his wife and wondering how he could ever put up with a woman with such an awkward nose, the woodcutter said: "I'll try." Grasping the string of sausages, he tugged with all his might. But he simply pulled his wife over on top of him. The pair sat on the floor, gazing sadly at each other.

"What shall we do now?" they said, each thinking the same thought.

"There's only one thing we can do ..." ventured the woodcutter's wife timidly.

"Yes, I'm afraid so." her husband sighed, remembering their dreams of riches, and he bravely wished the third and last wish "I wish the sausages would leave my wife's nose."

And they did. Instantly, husband and wife hugged each other tearfully, saying "Maybe we'll be poor, but we'll be happy again!"

That evening, the only reminder of the woodcutter's meeting with the elf was the string of sausages. So the couple fried them, gloomily thinking of what that meal had cost them.

So, be ultra careful about wishing your future...

Your personal heroine:

One other thing, do please look inside you for your personal heroine or hero. Male or female. Fantasy or real. Most people at one time or another have had a figure that they would like to model themselves on. Look at yours. Don't have one? Then dig back in your past, you are bound to find one. When you have found this model, look at her and try to figure out if she's a good role model for living in the here and now. If the answer is yes you don't need to look further. You have found your companion. Your fantasy companion whom you can involve in your constant, yes constant, struggle to live in the present.

When would you like to start glowing? If, as I suspect, you said now, then you are indeed clever, there is no time but the present.

G = go for it

L = love it

O = open your self

W = with your whole being

glowglow
glowglow
glowglow
glowglow
glowglow

13 SOME PEOPLE GLOW

Reflections on the First Time.

My paternal grandmother was over 90 years of age as I visited her about six months after she went to life with her daughter and her son in law, my aunt and uncle. For the first time in her life she was in bed because of illness. It was also the first time that I experienced a person being completely translucent. Amazing. It was as if there was a flood-light inside her and she emanated a glow that was truly wonderful. It seemed to illuminate the whole room and set off a chain of warm feelings inside me. Up to this point I had always experienced this grandmother as being cold, strict and unapproachable. In fact years later I got confirmation on this point from many people who knew her... she really was a cold bitch!

However, on this particular day, in this particular time, she was glowing. It was a great experience for me and when she died a few months later I was grateful to have had the opportunity of being with her in this state of glow.

It overshadowed all the previous unpleasantness that I associated with her.

Lesson No.1; it is never too late to glow.

I was 18 when I had this first hand experience of a glowing person and it was many years later before I experienced it again. It was nevertheless significant for me because it gave me a benchmark for glow and glowing. As children or teenagers we do, in general, tend to be more open although it does seem that the age of innocence is progressively shorter as the progress of industrialised culture and civilisation becomes faster and faster.

Try remembering your days at school. Which teachers do you remember? What was it about them that made them live on in your memory?

Do experiences in adulthood influence glow? Lets first have a look at glow in the work place. A professor at the London Business School, Lynda Gratton, has done a lot of research into the question of how to 'stay ahead of the curve' in the world of big business. She and her colleagues have designed programmes to teach people how to learn about being extrovert, how to actively seek cooperation and conversation within the network of people they have or would like to have business dealings with. They then go on to explore how to learn from these people. Finally there are programmes designed to spark off the potential energy that is often locked in within those people who are ambitious about being successful in the world of big business. For me personally, they tend to concentrate too much on things like 'will power', 'positive thinking' and other mainly rational and cognitive methodologies. Not really up my street, but if you are ambitious and want to get along in the corporate world, you might want to look more into these methods.

My early experience in the corporate world as a young successful manager in the business of organising and promoting trade fairs (my last assignment was to conceive and design the trade and cultural exhibition to commemorate the Investiture of Prince Charles as Prince of Wales.), taught me primarily that it would not be good for my health to carry on. You can imagine that living on half a bottle of whisky and seventy cigarettes a day as a near thirty year old is not necessarily a good recipe for a long and healthy life!

Maybe I was full of a kind of 'business glow' in those days, but I decided to turn my back on that world, to start again by studying natural therapy in the UK and Eastern Europe, became a Naturopath, trained in Group Encounter, and studied analytical psychology at the C. G. Jung Institute in Zurich, before opening a private psychotherapy practice in Frankfurt, Germany where I worked for more than 25 years.

After 'dropping out' of the business world I started to explore the spiritual world; during my forays into Buddhism I enrolled in a series of lectures at the Buddhist Society in London and, through that, got to know about meditation. Which in turn led me to an experience which I can only describe as an 'inner glow', which then led me to become a Quaker.

Nowadays I think of glowing as more of an internal process but the important thing is that you end up glowing rather than being burned out at the end of the process, whether you approach it from an extrovert or an introvert perspective.

Can teachers help you glow? There was a marvellous Swiss educationist called Jean Piaget who was the first to point out how important it is to learn by making mistakes rather than by constantly trying to be right. Think about it. One way to learn is by drill, just like you learn in the army by doing exactly what you are told. The other way is by making mistakes and learning through the personal relationship between your experiences and ideas. Piaget was the founder of the constructivist theory of teaching and learning.

We all know people or children who are so afraid of making a mistake that they end up doing nothing at all. Very rarely would we describe them as glowing personalities.

Do film stars automatically glow? Glow and Stardom are two different things. All stars glow but only at a distance. The same thing applies to film stars. All film stars glow at a distance but only some of them glow if you are close. Since the 'paparazzi' came on the scene, even film stars are not safe from being exposed as also being human. I personally do not know many film stars, but over the years I have met a number of actors. Some of them certainly have some sort of inner energy that manifests in the form of a radiant glow that probably lies at the root of what is known as stage presence. Lighting and make-up can certainly help to make an actor stand out on stage but are certainly no substitute for a glow that comes from deep within the person. One can certainly learn various techniques that can help make the most of the various positive traits that everyone has, whether it is learning to speak clearly in a way that is pleasing for the ear or even in just learning to keep still, when addressing an audience of guests at a wedding or a class of fellow students.

Have you ever heard a glow on the radio? During the early part of July 2012, in Margate, Kent in Southern England, 120 people had a 'glow and sound' experience. It was during the course of an art exhibition at Limbo Sub Station, where the photographer Edda Jones and the sound artist Russell Burden created a 'Sensory Installation in Darkness', called Close to Darkness. To quote from the press release of the Arts Council England funded project:

'Close to Darkness is a collaborative exploration of duality and polarity, ranging from the interface between lightness & darkness and positive & negative, to the realm of the seen & unseen and the heard & unheard , in an immersive installation work.'

Working in the mediums of photography and sound, Edda Jones and Russell Burden are seeking to create a sensory experience in a darkened space. The participants enter near total darkness and are enveloped in a cloud of sound. A sharpening of their senses will then help to slowly discover the faintly glowing still images on the walls – revealing themselves fully as the eyes grow accustomed to the darkness. Symbolic cues to highlight the mystery of light and dark; the alchemical wonder of the photographic process mirroring that of retinal translation – underpinned by a careful study of abstraction. All the while, the site-specific sound piece will continue and introduce another layer of sensory understanding.'

Here we learn that glowing is a slow process. You have to let it slowly develop in order to get the full and powerful impact, particularly if you are coming into the darkness from the light. One could also extrapolate and say that in order to connect with the inner glow, one has to slowly move into the darker realms of the unconscious mind. Which sometimes means confronting things that make one anxious. Which brings us back to yet another connection between worry and glow.

Celtic culture has always been into alchemical processes, whether smelting of ore to make metal or the role of glowing fires to greet both the onset of Spring as well as preparing for the Winter seasons. It is therefore no coincidence that illuminated manuscripts have played an important historical role in the interface of words and paper. The words are 'illuminated' by the glowing colours, and especially by the gold. In modern Wales there are numerous local festivals celebrating the literary and musical arts, culminating in an annual literary and musical festival called the National Eisteddfod where the two best writers get rewarded by, a crown for free verse and a chair for a poem in strict metre. You can be sure that the winning writers will glow when their names are announced.

Celebrities and glowing. Now that is a very interesting topic. Do they glow because they are celebrities or are they celebrities due to their ability to glow? A little story about my experiences with two celebrities may help to clarify. During a public occasion in a foreign country I was seated next to a very prim looking fellow, whom I said hello to and introduced myself to by name. He looked down his nose and said… nothing! So I said, "And who are you?" upon which he drew himself up in his chair and announced, rather than said, "I am the ******* ambassador!", naming one of the major nations, and then completely ignored me for the rest of the evening. Later on, talking to friends, they explained to me that he was probably deeply offended that I did not recognise him, because he appeared on TV every other day and was obviously working very hard to be a celebrity. He was definitely not a glowing person as far as I was concerned. Coincidentally or not, he was replaced soon after.

Many years ago, soon after I went to live and work in Germany, I was invited to a dinner party and introduced to a very attractive and glowing woman Hannelore Elsner, whom, I later found out, was a celebrated film star. There is no question in my mind that her glowing personality had a great deal to do with her stardom.

Going on holiday is often very conducive to putting a glow on your cheeks, particularly if it's a winter sports holiday. Unfortunately this type of glowing is somewhat short lived. But the good news is that an improved level of physical health really manifests itself in an improvement of skin quality, which in turn helps to communicate any inner glowing that you have.

When do we stop learning? Some people never stop learning and some people never even start learning. Or at least they never start learning from their mistakes. And that really is what learning is all about. Everyone makes mistakes but not everyone is interested in learning from their mistakes. That also applies to glowing. Even if you were glowing all the time when you were a little baby, the chances are that the glow started to diminish as you grew up. Or even later. Or even earlier. Let's assume that you could do with a bit more glow in your life.

It is never too late to start opening up. It is never to late to take risks. It is never too late to learn. So, don't worry, start glowing!

How can younger people learn to glow? There are no secrets about glowing. Like learning most things, we have to start off with information or knowledge, then start practising and ultimately combine the knowledge and the practical experience and before you know it, you are glowing and, most importantly, the people around you will notice. They will say things like; 'What have you been doing, you look great', or they might just smile at you.

Do dead people glow? What a strange question, but you are hopefully used to being asked strange questions by now. Just try going into a church that has paintings or icons and you will find lots of dead people being pictured with a glowing halo around their head, the old symbol for saintliness or holiness.

Sometimes you will see teenagers, both male and female, who positively glow with life and energy, whereas others have already started the process of fading away.

Advertisements often picture sexy looking people as being glowing as if trying to convey a secret form of magnetism that draws people to them.

In the same sort of way successful people are often portrayed as being a glowing success. However there is an interesting phenomena which I would like to label 'intrinsic glow': that is the glow that comes from within the person, irrespective of power, of office or any of those trappings of power. But then there is another side and that is what I call 'extrinsic glow': the power that comes with an office, a role, or even a brand. Think pop stars, film stars, politicians, Apple. We have often heard stars talking about the freedom for them of being in a society where they are unknown, where they can be a normal person, i.e. without the artificial glow that usually surrounds them and that of course attracts a lot of attention and forced intimacy which can sometimes be threatening.

There is also a darker side of extrinsic glow: the glow that comes with corrupted power. The kind of glow that we have often seen, that is constructed around such powerful people as Hitler or Stalin or indeed all dictators. The key word is 'constructed'. The main tool used to construct this type of glow is propaganda, where images and symbols of real or perceived success are linked directly to the person with the power. We have all seen pictures of ordinary people completely distraught at news of the death of a dictator responsible for the deaths of untold innocent persons whose only crime was that they were in the way.

You might well think that is so obvious I don't have to make such a big deal of it. Yes and no. As far as publicly known dictators are concerned, you are right, there is no need to. However there are lots of people out there who are constantly trying to use their own corrupted power for their own ends. You might be well advised to look out for them.

Poverty can sometimes be glowing, particularly if you are a saint called Francis of Assisi, otherwise poor people are often perceived as having lost their shine, particularly in our increasingly material and wealth oriented 'advanced' societies.

One of the most amazing sights that I ever saw was driving through Rajasthan, India in the 1990s and seeing a woman building a wall with sun-dried bricks. She was dressed in a pink and blue sari, had rolled up her sleeves to the elbow, was using her bare hands to scoop up and spread a mud-like mortar, and laying the bricks at quite a fast pace. Marvellous and beautiful. Whether she felt an inner glow is another matter, but she certainly gave me a great and glowing cross-cultural experience!

Have rich people got an increased chance to glow? In an extroverted, superficial way it is relatively easy to get a surface glow with money. Cosmetics, clothes and perfume can, with a bit of help from a professional stylist, create, at least from a distance, an aura of glow. It's only when you are really close that you can begin to see that it is just on the surface and that it really has nothing at all to do with the real person inside.

Hopefully I do not need to stress that the glow we are talking about in this book has very little in common with the glow that you can shop for.

Glow and politics is a very interesting field and it seems to me that it is mostly a sort of fringe phenomena. When a new political movement is beginning to form itself there is often a lot of enthusiasm around, which in turn, leads often to a general spirit of excitement, even adventure, the start of an adventurous journey hopefully towards a new world, a new state, a new order. Not many people can keep this up after the goal has been attained. But there have always been people like Mahatma Ghandi in India, Nelson Mandela in Africa, or Aung San Suu Kyi in Burma who keep on glowing and inspiring for decades. I think I am probably right to assume that you, my reader, will agree with me that the three human beings mentioned above are good and wonderful people who gave and give their life to good and honourable causes and deserve our respect and gratitude.

However there have been others around too. People like Adolf Hitler, Pol Pot, General Pinochet and others. Many, many people were attracted to these men and continued to support them while awful things were happening all around them. Why? Have you ever seen any of these or other leaders of movements that are generally classified nowadays as tyrannous, evil or anti-human rights or whatever, just basically not good, on TV or film? Did you notice the enthusiasm, even love that their supporters expressed towards them? It does seem to indicate that charisma, in the sense of a compelling attractiveness that inspires devotion in others, can be used in the cause of good or bad depending on the character or personality of the leader.

While it is not difficult to find men and women, either living or dead who lead movements for good or bad, it is extremely difficult to find women that could be classified as tyrants or dictators. The nearest I got was with the following two women who did not rule on their own but seemed to have used the power of their husbands to realise their own, often bad and evil, plans. Margaret Honecker in East Germany whom I saw in a German TV interview around 2012 came over as arrogant and unsympathetic, and Elena Ceauşescu the wife of the Romanian dictator deposed in 1989. They were both subjects of propaganda campaigns to make them into ideal 'Mother of the Nation' even though, by all accounts, the two of them did not demonstrate the type of qualities that we would normally associate with a good, caring and loving mother.

The word recreation has an interesting look about it if we split it up, re and creation. Try to make time in your own life to re-create your capacity for glowing. You surely won't regret it.

id

14 MIND & GLOW

**A short Introduction to the Roots
of Humanistic Psychology.**

What was so special about the Druids? Were the Druids
into glowing? Well, they were certainly into fire and light
and, in the same way as the Celts were one of the first
peoples to discover how to transmute metals through fire,
the Druids were interested in the process of the oak tree
transmuting into mistletoe. Did you know that it is impossible to see with the naked eye at what point the mistletoe
growing out of the oak tree becomes mistletoe and not
oak? For the Druids the mistletoe was a holy plant, maybe
because it represents mankind emerging from the earth
mother and still being attached to the earth and nature.
The kind of glowing we are dealing with, is the glow that
comes from being close to the natural you. Being close
to the real you. Being close to the appropriate you. Being
close to the authentic you. Being close to your Self. Being
close to the original you. And so on and so forth, I'm sure
you know by now what I mean.

In this chapter, we will be exploring various ways that people and cultures have devised to attain this desirable state of glowing, of emanating and radiating what has, from time to time, being called joie de vivre, life force, phlogistin, chi, vital force, orgone or just energy.

What influence did the Chinese yellow emperor have? A few hundred years BC saw the first definitive written codex of Chinese medicine, usually known under the name of the mythical Yellow Emperor. Of particular interest to us is the reference to the best time for diagnosing a patient. It's the time of the first glow of the sun after the dark of the night. They had the experience of being able to feel the pulse at this particular time and to ascertain whether the patient was moving towards life or death or just simply static. One of the fundamental principles of the time was that of a universal life energy or 'chi', the state of which was the basis for any treatment.

Going back even further in time, to around 1400 BC, we find the Oracle of Delphi where a priestess of Apollo gave predictions, usually in exchange for gold offerings. At that time, the Temple was perceived as the navel of the world, symbolised by an eternally burning flame in the sacred shrine in the centre of the temple.

The Egyptians on the other hand, even further back in time, saw the sun as being the one creator, the one god that determines everything, so life was based on keeping him/it/her, happy and peaceful. A time when the glow of the sun dying every evening and the glow of the new sun being born every single morning was a constant reminder of the fragility of the individual and of the importance of having knowledgeable priests to make sure that the sun, the god and the Pharaoh were kept alive and happy.

It was during the time of the ancient Egyptians that the

first painted halo around a human head in a piece of art appeared, probably a play on the glowing aura around the sun.

This was the time when gold, with it's constant glow if light played on it, was in great favour with the managers of the god industry. It was often used to dazzle people. Sounds familiar?

It took quite a while in the western part of the earth before Aesclupius started to look at the dreams of his patients for some kind of clue as to the type of treatment that would heal the individual.

However, pictorial representations of the gods of ancient Greece and Rome were often shown with a halo around their heads.

But we have to travel further East to find further references to the role of glowing in life processes. Asian art, as it has developed within both Hindu and Buddhist traditions, often shows fire and light emanating from the whole body or human figure, not just the head.

Christian art often depicts it's saints and heroes with a halo around their head in the same manner as previous Roman artists pictured their gods.

Artistic depictions of holiness in African art do not appear to focus on haloes apart from, of course, various Christian uses of glow around persons. However, glowing stars have an important part in various ancient myths.

Whilst Victorian England was fighting glow even to the extent of covering the polished wooden legs of pianos because of the morally perceived danger of any associations with the glow of the healthy human body, continental Europe, in the form of people like Sigmund Freud and Carl Jung, was experimenting with releasing glowing dreams of liberating sexuality and sensuality from the shackles of restrictive social and cultural moral opinions.

Wilhelm Reich was a young medical doctor when he first made contact with Freud and Psychoanalysis, at a time when Freud was established as an authority in his field. Reich soon got into trouble with his colleagues when he started to talk about such way-out concepts as a 'universal life energy'. When he lectured about the possibility of actually physically touching and massaging his female and male patients whilst dressed only in underclothes, he was thrown out of the International Psychoanalytic Society. After some time in Scandinavia, where he trained a few colleagues, Reich moved to the United States, trained a handful of medical therapists, got into trouble with the Food and Drug Administration for his work with Orgone Life Energy and by all accounts, died a broken man.

It took many years before Wilhelm Reich was recognised as the Founding Father of all present day body-oriented forms of psychotherapy and his writings on youth, on sexuality and on social and individual repression, was an inspiration for many during the time of the sexual revolution of the 1960s.

Two of his students, John Pierrakos and Alexander Lowen developed his ideas during the late 1950s into what became known as Bioenergetics, before a split between the two founders, after which John Pierrakos went on to develop Core Therapy, together with Eva Pierrakos.

I was introduced to John by his new wife Eva after meeting her at a party in London in the late 1960s and later, I met Ilse Ollendorf Reich, the widow of Wilhelm Reich, at a Quaker conference in Germany in the 1990s.

Once upon a time in the Black Forest area of Germany, in Baden Baden in the time up to 1934, there lived and worked a quite extraordinary man called Georg Groddeck. A German physician and naturopath, he was a lonely pioneer in the field of psychosomatic medicine for decades, combining natural therapies such as massage and hydrotherapy with psychoanalysis.

He placed great emphasis on the condition of the skin. A skin glowing with vitality and health was a very positive sign.

He was also one of the very few people who influenced Sigmund Freud rather that the other way round. Groddeck's ideas expressed in his book titled 'The Book of the Id' inspired Freud to develop the concept of the 'Id' in The Ego and the Id.

A modern day representative of the glowing tradition of both Reich and Groddeck was Gerda Boyesen whom I befriended in London during the 1960s and 1970s. She was visiting us one day and happened to overhear me speaking on the phone to my mother in my 'mother tongue' – Welsh. Gerda was overjoyed and said something like, "How wonderful, I have just heard your true spirit, your Id!"

Even though Groddeck and Jung had no contact, or at least there is no contact documented, they both approached illness as a problem of the whole person rather than a collection of independent symptoms, an approach which they shared with Wilhelm Reich. An approach that, to this day, is still not recognised in mainstream medicine.

However, in 1982 John Conger wrote a book about Jung and Reich exploring what might have happened if they had met! Because they never did meet.

Years later in 2004, John Conger reviewing his work, wrote the following...

"In reading new brain research, I have been struck with how much Reich would have resonated to this work. In (1999) The Feeling of What Happens: Body and Emotion in the Making of Consciousness. (New York: Harcourt, Inc.), Antonio Damasio talks about the intelligence and function of a single cell and its innate mechanisms for survival. Damasio, like Reich and other present day neuroscientists, conceive mind, self and consciousness as an integrated biological construct, and they pursue an evolutionary tale concerning our vulnerable humanity with compassion and excitement. Damasio writes:

"A simple organism made up of one single cell, say, an amoeba, is not just alive but bent on staying alive. Being a brainless and mindless creature, an amoeba does not know of its own organism's intentions in the sense that we know of our equivalent intentions. But the form of an intention is there, nonetheless, expressed by the manner in which the little creature manages to keep the chemical profile of its internal milieu in balance while around it, in the environment external to it, all hell may be breaking loose."(p. 136)"

There is also current research in sub-atomic physics, which explores the relationship between energy and material, so who knows what will happen in the future?

Interestingly enough, although Acupuncture has increasingly established itself as a mainstream medical treatment for pain reduction, etc. the underlying theoretical concept of life energy is still not at all recognised in orthodox medical circles when it comes to establishing possible treatments in the realm of psychotherapy and of psycho-somatic medicine, where the dominant thinking is still based on the split between body and mind.

Interestingly enough, a possible source of future therapeutic development is to be found in the multi-discipline research into the treatment of civilians and soldiers traumatised by war.

Unfortunately, there is much more money and material available for research into weapons for war as opposed to treating the aftermath of war.

stop

look

listen

15 MIND & WORRY

Labels, Methods, Techniques.

Are drugs of any use in combating worry? This is of course a question that's been around as long as worry itself. Probably the most simple answer is 'yes'. There are many kinds of drugs around, medicinal as well as recreational, which can be and often are, used to divert one's attention to something other than worry. The most common example is alcohol. Then there are very sophisticated psycho-pharmaceutical drugs that steer processes away from the fears and anxieties that often accompany worries.

Common to all of these drugs is that they have no effect whatsoever on the root cause of the worry. They deal more or less effectively with the symptoms or side-effects of worry.

Worry itself is, under certain circumstances, manageable. The first step is to define the worry. The problem with taking drugs is that they tend to affect your perceptions, including your perception or awareness of the worry.

So, if you really want to learn about your worries you have to get to know them and the most direct way is without drugs. At this point I have to introduce a caveat: if you are in psychotherapeutic or psychiatric treatment with psycho-pharmaceutical drugs, DO NOT stop using the drugs before discussing it with your practitioner.

The use of hypnosis does indeed fall within the traditional definition of natural therapy but since my experience of it in the clinical context is very limited I will limit my commentary to suggesting that even though self-hypnosis can be extremely effective in, let's say hiding pain, it is not something I can recommend for dealing with worry since it simply makes the cause of the worry not available to the conscious mind and is therefore not very useful if one wants to explore the root cause of the thing that one is worried about.

Let us establish a working hypothesis that, buried more or less deep in our unconscious mind, is the key or root cause of our worries. Then the next step must surely be to explore this intimate area of our being. This is one explanation of why the healing temples of Asklepius, particularly the one in Epidaurus in ancient Greece, was so successful that it brought untold riches to the town. The patient had to sleep in the holy temple and the next day reported to his priest/healer the details of his dreams. The elements of the dream were analysed and the treatment was then prescribed according to the interpretation of the patient's dreams by the healer.

How then could it be that the dreams helped to find the root cause of the patient's malaise? There is really no short answer to this question. The only way to really learn about it, is to experience it in the hands of a therapist used to working with the appropriate tools. Let me give an example of how it works.

Jack, a young man, came to my consulting room complaining about his difficulty in not being able to sleep if lying on his back. He could not even lie down to relax on his back. He even woke up if he happened to move into this position at night. After some months of therapy he had a series of dreams centred around a temple culminating in a nightmarish dream where he was lying on a sacrificial altar in a huge temple all alone and woke up in a state of terror and anxiety. Eventually, it turned out that he was treated in a hospital at the age of two years for a suspected case of a highly infectious tropical disease. He spent three weeks in an isolation ward all alone before it became clear it was a false alarm. After working through the various emotional feelings from the perspective of a small baby, where, for example, a single hospital room would appear to be a huge hanger type of building, my client slowly started to feel comfortable and relaxed whilst lying on his back and soon was even able to sleep whilst lying on his back.

We have been looking at various ways of managing or treating worry and it is possible that you are beginning to wonder about the difference between worry, anxiety and depression. Well, you are not alone because the boundaries between these various states are quite flexible and are usually based on factors such as quality and quantity. For example, if I spend a lot of time in artificial sun studios getting a Hollywood tan and then worry about skin cancer, then that would be very realistic and not at all pathological. If, on the other hand, I am a night worker and start to worry about going out during the day if the sun is shining, based upon reading some article about the dangers of sunbathing, then that is not at all realistic and one would be justified in thinking this is someone with an anxiety syndrome who could possibly benefit from seeing a psychotherapist. And, finally, if this same night shift worker stays in bed all day without going out at all, we would be justified in thinking that this person could well be suffering from clinical depression.

It is important to differentiate between worry and concern. A concern is usually a real problem or conflict that needs to solved or resolved. So, if you find yourself caught up in worrying about something, stop for a minute and ask yourself: Is there a real answer to this problem even if I myself am not aware of it or am I worrying about something that is either abstract or fantasy such as: 'If the football team that I support loses the next game, nothing will ever go right in my life'. A concern is something like: 'If I fail my driving test I will not get the job as a truck driver'. Of course, it's pretty obvious in this instance that passing the driving test is very much influenced by the time and energy I have invested in learning about driving, whereas my learning about football will certainly not affect the performance of the team I am a fan of.

Rather than looking for the newest, best, more progressive technique, it is sometimes worthwhile to stop and look at the practitioner. Sometimes it is preferable to be treated by a good therapist using the 'wrong' technique as opposed to be treated using a 'right' technique from a not so good therapist. Try trusting your own feelings when you first meet the therapist. Does she make you feel welcome and at ease or is your reaction to her person more in the direction of being intimidated and feeling uneasy.

One useful rule is to wait a bit. If, after 20 minutes, you still do not feel comfortable with the therapist, if you cannot conceive of being really open, you may well be better off looking somewhere else. But try expressing your discomfort before you go any further.

The therapist may react in a way that could be beneficial

for you. It's always worth a try! As regards which method or technique is best for treating a worry that is beginning to become a chronic problem, we can well apply this question to any problem that calls for any kind of psychotherapeutic treatment. It is possible to trace the development of modern psychotherapy back to the late 19th century where 'Coueism' and 'Mesmerism' began to appeal to people as a way for them to more or less consciously influence the course of their illness. Then came Sigmund Freud and the enormous theoretical production through him and his increasing followers. The next step was a splitting off by such persons as Carl Gustav Jung, Alfred Adler, Wilhelm Reich and others, some of whom in turn gathered followers so that by the middle of the 20th century it was difficult, for an outsider, to differentiate between the various schools. Added to that, there developed, parallel to the depth-psychological schools the concept of behavioural psychology, which in turn led to behavioural therapy. Not to mention such methods as 'cognitive-rational', emotive, gestalt, body-oriented, encounter and so on.

In the 21st century there have been other changes. Life coaching, counselling, coaching are some of the words that are more common nowadays. Again, my advice is to use your own experience and your own judgement as to how you feel during the first 20 minutes of being with your new practitioner, whether she is an orthodox medical specialist, a psychologist, or a Mongolian shaman. It is, after all, your own mind, your own soul and your own spirit, let alone your own body. It is your duty and your responsibility, always assuming, dear reader that you are over the age of 18 years!

The psycho-pharmaceutical industry has often tended to try to develop medication that will create new markets for their production facilities, just like any other industry.

It may well be a good idea to talk to someone before you look for a person who can write you a prescription.

body
rock

16 WORRY AND THE BODY

Who would have thought the body can worry?

What happens when I have difficulty swallowing? You've probably heard someone saying, "I just could not swallow it" referring to a far-fetched story that someone told. Now, if I have something that I am worried about but don't want to face, the worry may well affect my whole digestive system leading from the feeling of having a lump in my throat to having a constipated bowel.

One of the most common disorders amongst female teenagers in the western world is anorexia and the related bulimia. Anorexia has to do with being so worried about getting fat that you stop eating, whereas bulimia represents the act of vomiting, again to prevent one getting fat although sometimes mixed up with worries about the harmful effect of the foods digested.

So, eating disorders are often associated with worry and or anxiety. We even sometimes say, "Oh, that is difficult for me to digest!" Between my mouth and my guts is my stomach. The stomach is a very sensitive organ and reacts strongly to worries particularly if they are accompanied by anxiety related to the worry.

Does the heart betray feelings? Many cultures associate the heart with feelings of love. Anyone who has experienced being in love knows that this can often lead to unpleasant side effects. For instance, when the loved one does not reply to an email or a phone-call. Then the heart starts to beat quicker and can even lead to an uncomfortably tight feeling in the chest area.

It was not long ago that one spoke about someone having a 'nervous breakdown'. It is no longer used in a medical diagnostic sense but it might be interesting to look at the dictionary definition. According to the Oxford Dictionary: The noun describes a period of mental illness resulting from severe depression, stress, or anxiety. In practice that means that there is a danger if worry escalates into anxiety and then this state continues for a longer period of time, leading to a break-down of vital systems in the body.

Nowadays it is widely recognised that bodily exercise is a good thing. What is not so widely accepted is that it is also important as a preventative measure. As a prophylactic against not only diseases affecting the joints or the muscles but also illnesses associated with the mind and the soul/spirit.

Most fitness studios these days have a 'cardio programme'. Give it a try; it may not give you a muscular body but it might well give you an enhanced feeling of well-being.

Ever felt the hair at the back of your neck bristling? Well, it could be a side effect of goose bumps, sometimes known as goose pimples, when the muscles under the skin contract to make your hairs stand on end. We can look at goose bumps as a sort of skin orgasm as a result of an emotional climax. It can be triggered off by various emotional feelings from fear to admiration and, most importantly, cannot be faked!

What do you reply to the following question: "Are you angry?" Do you tend to go on the defensive and say, 'No' because you're afraid to admit it? Well, how do we know that we are angry, what are the signs we can look for? Firstly, there is your heart beat: it gets faster with increasing anger, then breathing tends to maximise, together with increasing muscle tension, often around the shoulders, even reaching down into the hands and leading to clenched fists. Stomach muscles can spasm, your face can feel hot. There are many signs there, if you are prepared to accept the possibility of being angry. Acceptance of anger is the first step in being able to do something to manage it. If you are not willing to acknowledge anger in the first instance you run into the danger of it escalating and possibly leading to you hurting yourself or others.

Clench your teeth and fight on, is what the soldiers or, more often, their officers used to say during the first Word War. The problem was that many soldiers suffered from shell-shock and had to be hospitalised for treatment because they were unable to cope. Fear is a very real emotional feeling and modern soldiers are often taught how to deal with it before they have to deal with being under fire. But there is obviously room for improvement; there are still far too many veteran soldiers suffering from traumatic stress related disorders in Germany, UK and in the USA. In fact the problem of post traumatic stress disorders has led to major health issues amongst ex-soldiers, including many suicide deaths. There are even some statistics that seem to show that more veterans die through suicide than active soldiers on the battlefield. Of course statistics can be used to prove almost anything, but nevertheless there is an increasing body of evidence that stress in times of battle affects not only the civilian population but is a serious health hazard for active soldiers.

Fear and worry, and the effect of fear and worry not only on one's self but also on others is a very complex theme. One day in my practice in Frankfurt, Germany a woman came to see me. She was a dentist and had to stop working because the fear and anxieties of her patients had so affected her that she could no longer treat them. Now most of us can feel sympathy with people being afraid of dental treatment, but how many think about the possible effect on the dentist?

Is there a connection between constipation and feeling? Wilhelm Reich was one of the first to point out the central role of the gastrointestinal tract in most of the symptoms associated with the term 'psychosomatic'. Gerda Boyesen proceeded to develop a whole therapeutic system around this phenomena.

Why do little kids pee in their pants? Haven't we all, at some point or another, had the feeling of 'wetting my pants'? The bladder is a very sensitive organ not only in elderly men with a prostate problem.

There is a strange phenomena which I like to label 'genetic memory' even though it is not, strictly speaking, anything directly to do with our genes. Think of it as a shorthand symbol for our ability to absorb experiences from our parents or even our grandparents without these experiences being verbally expressed in our presence. A rather more orthodox term is 'trans-generational emotional experience'.

The horrific untold stories of a father's war experiences. The mother's trauma of childhood abuse. Such experiences can sometimes affect the following generations.

Sonya suffered from time to time from nightmares. After many months of analytical work she started to do some inner family research, found that her grandmother was brutally raped at the end of the second World War, was able to work through this information and eventually enjoyed going to sleep without worrying about having nightmares.

Because of the work of people like Eric Kandel, the Nobel Science Prize recipient, we now know that memory affects the brain structure but the theme of unconsciously transmitted memories is a field where very little research has been published, even though the area of war induced trauma is slowly moving into the realm of public consciousness.

What do rapid eye movements have to do with worry? There is a whole new therapy form based on rapid eye movements. Sometimes people turn to hypnotism for relief from worry. If you are worried for instance about going to the dentist and your worries are so great that you do not even go for a check up it would probably be a good idea to look for a dentist who practices hypnotherapy, it could well bring you relief as well as healthy teeth.

On the other hand, if you tend to worry about more intangible things and they prevent you from sleeping or concentrating on your work you might well benefit from psychotherapy.

Are you a good in soldiering on? Basically, one can say with some degree of certainty that a body glowing with good health can help one be mobile and physically active when worries start to be chronic and start to infiltrate one's consciousness to the extent of trying to persuade one to just forget about washing today or to stay in bed this morning. If you are basically fit and in good shape you

have a good chance to kick yourself in the bum and go out
and do your thing rather than slide in to a state that could
lead to depression. And nobody wants that! The image
of the ideal warrior comes up quite often both in Eastern
spiritual and religious writings as well as in Western myths
and, let's not forget the Salvation Army who are still doing
a non-romantic but often very effective type of social work
amongst the disenfranchised minorities all over the world
that hardly ever gets publicity but has still helped millions
of people.

Sometimes it's important just to look after your physical
body, particularly when your mind starts to invest too
much energy in exploring things for you to worry about.

fast

17 BODY & GLOW

Healthy mind, healthy body and all that jazz.

The legendary fountain of youth is a secret spring, the water of which, when drunk, has the potential of giving you eternal youth, with all the attendant benefits such as beauty, attractiveness and health, even glowing health as opposed to the common type of health. Where do I find it? What is it, where is it and how does it work?

That, of course, is the question that has preoccupied people for thousands of years. Herodotus looked for it in Ancient Greece, Alexander the Great searched for it, even the legendary Yellow Emperor was interested in it 5000 years ago in China.

So, we can say with some certainty that the possibility of discovering a secret spring that can give you everlasting youth has always fascinated people, just think about Cleopatra and her bath of milk.

Well, I have news for you. You will certainly not achieve

eternal life, you will not experience a journey back in time, but you might well feel better, your skin will certainly feel better and, who knows, you might end up feeling more beautiful and attractive!

Sounds good?

Water. What? Water is the secret. Yep, just drink ordinary clean water, either from the tap if you have a good drinking water mains supply, from a bottle or even from a mountain spring if you are lucky enough to live in places like Snowdonia in Wales or in the Swiss mountain countryside.

It's very simple but not very easy. You see you have to ONLY drink water, and that for a few days!

Of course you can start slowly... try just one day of drinking only water and eating or drinking nothing else. Some people find it exciting and see it as a great adventure. Others find it extremely difficult. And you? There is only one way to find out. Try it!

BUT, make sure that you are in a normal state of health and not taking any medicines. NB This is very important.

What has air got to do with glowing? Do you watch a lot of sport? Then you will have noticed that some athletes really seem to have a glow around them, usually if the sport involves a lot of deep breathing. Yoga has always focussed on the importance of deep and regular breathing and even those of you who do not even like sports will have probably experienced a nice glowing inside feeling after a brisk country walk, particularly if there were some hills to be climbed.

Glowing is of course both a very personal and intimate bodily feeling that produces reactions ranging from embarrassment to ecstasy, and can also be used to describe a more or less objective state of being that can be noted by others, even though 'glow' is not in itself a strictly scientific term.

'Asian Glow' is the name of a skin complaint associated with incomplete metabolism of alcohol that seems to occur more often in Asian cultures. It describes a rather uncomfortable reaction to alcohol with such symptoms as reddening of skin on and around the face.

Needless to say, this is not the kind of glowing that we are concerned with here, even though it could be an interesting path to follow in terms of the power that alcohol has in present day society when the fact that a perfectly healthy body rejects alcohol is seen as a problem rather than a possibility to maybe look at the question of 'do I really need to drink alcohol?'.

In ancient Greece, successful athletes could accumulate riches just as much as today. So we can probably assume that the winners of the games then, whether in Olympia or not, were perfectly capable of glowing and basking in the glory of their success on the sport field.

Which brings us to a question that is right up to date. 'Can sport make me healthy?'. The answer is: 'It depends'. No, that's not a cop-out answer. There have always been people who used sport to push themselves and others over the top, over the barrier separating health-inducing movement and activity from potentially damaging things like doping to over-strained muscles and ligaments.

It's always been a question of balance. A balance between developing muscle strength on the one hand and stamina on the other, sprint and marathon. A classic illustration of the problem is to do with running, whether you call it jogging or anything else. Many people have ended up with damaged legs or feet or worse, through a combination of a running technique which makes you land on your heels (resulting in a recurring shock that is transmitted from heel to neck via legs, pelvis and spine) and buying shoes which are more and more upholstered.

The problem with the shoes that have thick soles, is that you lose the ability to feel the ground under your feet, whilst the technique that you use to run can be re-trained so that you land on the middle or on the ball of your foot as well as keeping an upright position.

That is what's behind the increasingly popular 'barefoot running style'. You don't necessarily have to run with no shoes but the difference you will feel by learning a new technique could well be a big surprise.

Sport and glowing have often been linked right from the very beginning of civilisation. Gold, the ultimate glowing metal, medals for the winner, a golden halo around the heads of the athletic gods, are just two examples of how intertwined they both are.

Meditate and glow? Really? Well, I am not sure that you will start to develop a halo or an aura around you if you start to meditate but I am quite sure that at some point you will start to feel a warm glow inside you if you per-severe with your practice. And that may well be reward enough.

We've written about halos as depicting a glow around the heads of gods, saints or holy people, but what do they actually mean? A halo, also called a nimbus, is a geometric shape, usually in the form of a disk, circle, ring, or rayed structure. Traditionally, the halo represents a radiant light around or above the head of a divine or sacred person. Since halos are found nowhere in the Bible, what is their origin in Christianity?

Interestingly, the word 'halo' comes from the Greek word for a threshing floor. It was on these floors that oxen moved round and round in a continuous circle on the ground, making a circular path in the shape we now associate with halos. Many ancient societies, including the Egyptians, Indians and Romans, used a circular sign to suggest supernatural forces, such as angels, at work.

In art, halos originally appeared as disks of gold sketched upon the head of a figure. This depicted a sphere of light radiating from the head of the person, suggesting that the subject was in a mystical state or sometimes, that the person was very smart. Because of its shape and colour, the halo was also associated with the sun and resurrection. By the fourth century, the halo had become widely used in standard Christian art. Essentially, it was used to mark a figure as being in the kingdom of light. Most commonly, Jesus and the Virgin Mary are shown with halos, along with the angels. In fact, halos are found in art forms all over the world. Sometimes, especially in the East, crowns are used instead of halos, but the meaning is the same: holiness, innocence and spiritual power.

One interesting question is whether Eastern glow represents an introverted type of glowing such as the inner glow described in various writing about meditation, whereas Western glow pictures a more extroverted type of glowing which is ably represented by the baroque style of art which used light in all its glory and was used primarily to promote the Roman Catholic Church.

Glow, Body and Sickness.

Welcome to the weird and wonderful world of Psyche and Soma, better known as Psychosomatic.

Most illnesses are experienced and felt as affecting your life, even the common cold is often a source of annoyance and irritation, sometimes triggering off fantasies of global pollution conspiracies or signalling the onset of some exotic disease.

Our capacity to imagine knows no bounds, the media is full of information about epidemics, new cancer scares. New medical developments are regularly proclaimed as being nearly miraculous only, a few sentences later, to be told that IF the tests are successful we MAY have found a cure that will be on the market in 5 or 10 years.

In many respects our world has become very mobile but as regards our attitude to being ill it has become more and more passive. Instead of reacting and going to our local medical practitioner when we feel ill, we tend more and more to put faith in screenings and tests to look for various possibilities that may mean that we could become ill in the future.

Instead of taking responsibility for our own health we have become passive and look for someone to tell us whether we are sick or not. With the increase of medical technology, the control of illness has passed from the patient to the doctor. One of the problems with this, is that most medical training nowadays is focussed on testing, labelling and medication and few medical students experience the possibility of seeing the patient as a real, human, person with hopes, fears, anxieties and so on.

The sad news is that a person who is ill, who is afraid, who is feeling lost, helpless and with no hope, is often regarded as being an irritating and stupid appendage of the known or unknown disease, and who is then often pressured to separate herself into a symptom part,the somatic, bodily part, which is then treated by an expert, and another, feeling part, the psyche or mind, which she has to deal with on her own. It sounds one-sided because it is!

Compliance and adherence are not just words; they represent a growing attitude amongst health practitioners, insurance schemes and companies, and health care providers, whether individuals or institutions. Comply, adhere to the plan. Do exactly what you are told, swallow the pills according to plan, don't question the expert. Shut up. In other words, behave as if you are a motor car, have your engine, mechanical and electronic parts regularly serviced and you'll keep on running until it's time to be replaced with the new, improved model.

Try thinking in terms of being your body as opposed to having a body, particularly when you find yourself being dissatisfied with a particular function. For example: instead of complaining about the virus that has just 'given' you a cold, try thinking about what you can do to increase your level of fitness, thus increasing your personal level of resistance to any bugs that are around.

Do you exercise? Regularly? If not, why not? Are you too young or too old, too fat or too thin, too tense or too relaxed, to energised or too lazy. What is your particular excuse?

Do you lack the motivation? Not many people recognise that their emotional life really governs their world. Try looking at the emotional feeling behind your attitude towards exercise. Try accepting the emotion and then look at it and check whether it is really appropriate for the situation you find yourself in today.

There was a very clever and very flamboyant financial adviser in the 1960s called, if I remember correctly, Bernie Cornfeld whose advertising slogan was: 'Do you sincerely want to be rich?'

Maybe you should try asking yourself the question: 'Do I sincerely want to have a body that glows with good health?' If not, that's perfectly OK with me! But if your answer is yes, then it might be a good idea to look for the cause of your not doing anything about getting there.

Some of us are very good about making plans, some of us are good at conceiving great projects, some of us are good at starting things, some of us are good at finishing things. What applies to you?

Maybe it's just time for you to start doing.

Have fun.

dreamy

edu-

ca-

tion

18 WORRY AND THE SOUL

A dip into the unconscious.

Does worry manifest itself in our dreams? During the last thirty-odd years of practising analytic psychotherapy I have indeed sometimes come across instances where a patient/client wakes up knowing the solution to a problem they had been worrying about. They had been worrying about the problem in the same way that a terrier dog 'worries' about a bit of cloth. Sometimes he throws it up in the air, takes it, growls at it, bites it, goes away, picks it up again, shakes his head at the same time as biting on the cloth, leaves it, goes away, comes back, starts the whole process all over again, etc.

It is conceivable that during our sleep our unconscious seems to be able to look at the problem in peace and quiet, sees a possible solution and when we wake up, there it is.

C. G. Jung's lifelong research into the various ways of being that mankind has explored, brought him into contact with the various paths we take during our own individual lives. He was convinced that the ultimate goal was to make contact with our own 'Self', the very core of our being on this earth.

On our way to the Self we, each one of us, has to go through various life processes, starting with being born and beginning the process of growing up. At this early stage of our life many of us accumulate various neuroses, ranging from the so-called 'normal neuroses' to complex neuroses developed as a result of traumatic experiences. If we progress more or less successfully through our teen-age years, then by the time we are 21 years of age we can usually look back at the things we worried about as a child and teenager with a little smile.

However, if things were not quite smooth, then quite often we enter adulthood with some worries which have been with us for so long that they have got lost in the back corners of our mind. These are the worries that are so 'normal' to us that we don't even consider them to be worries. Spend a minute thinking about your own life and just ask yourself if there are worries that are so much a part of your life that you have forgotten what it would be like without them. Think about it.

The spiritual life or the life of the spirit is an area that most people are clear about, whether they are interested in it or not. You, my dear reader, based on my working assumption, are someone who is at least open to the possibility that there is such a thing as a spiritual life which may well be of value to some. If so, the chances are that you have spent some time worrying or at least thinking about what role your soul/spirit has in your life. You may well be concerned about how to manage your time so that there is some space available for this aspect of your life. Do you even consider that in your time management procedures? Or do you just hope that you will, one day, find some time available for your spiritual life. Beware, you might be so busy that you will never find the time. What then?

Now that is really something worth worrying about!

Lots of people brought up in a religious community or environment, worry about sin, often in terms of how to avoid even thinking about the whole concept of sin and sinning, sometimes about the possible results of the sins that they personally have committed. In any case, it could well be very valuable for you to spend some time considering how relevant such concepts are for your present life and even lifestyle.

It might even be educational for you to consider what role the idea of sin, of you being 'bad', played in your early life, and whether it was ever used as an abuse of power that someone had over your life. Yes, abuse, or misuse of power is nowadays more and more recognised as being, unfortunately, part and parcel of many institutions, religious and others, as well as in too many families.

What guidelines do you have to help you decide what is right and what is wrong? Do you have any guidelines at all? Do you have a conscience? Do you have a god or a goddess or a godhead that you turn to for guidance on right and wrong, good or bad? How do you decide what to do in a difficult situation? Have you heard about those top managers in Switzerland who could not live with the hard and sometimes brutal atmosphere in their firm and who committed suicide because that was their only way out, in their opinion? Or about the young junior managers in China who took the same path for much the same reason? What has all that got to do with you and your life? What do think about societies where a few have so much money they really don't know what to do with it and a lot of people don't know where to get the money for an ice cream for their children?

Is it really true that it is easier for a camel to pass through a hole in a needle than it is for a rich person to go to heaven? What is heaven anyway? Is there such a thing? If so, is it somewhere on earth?

Is there such a thing as a good conscience, a bad conscience? Should we allow 12 or 13 year olds to drink alcohol to excess? Should we allow them to drink alcohol at all? Who is to say what is right? Should 14 year olds have sex? With 16 year olds? Or with 36 year olds? What are our guidelines in such matters?

Sometimes I think we should concentrate more on emotional education as opposed to the very rational kind of education that is mostly practiced. Would it not be useful to learn while at school how other people, grown up adults as well as children, deal with such things as worrying about things that could affect their life so much that their bad conscience tortures their whole future existence?

2013 saw a book published by the son of a famous Swiss psychoanalyst called Alice Miller. She became famous in the 1970s and 80s with her many books (including "The Drama of the Gifted Child"), about the traumatic upbringing of many generations of children in Europe, which she referred to as 'Black Pedagogy'. She quoted untold instances of child abuse long before the subject became notorious through instances of child abuse within the Roman Catholic Church. What came out in the book "Das wahre 'Drama des begabten Kindes'" ("The true 'Drama of the Gifted Child'".) by Martin Miller was the tragic truth that she herself was unable to break free from her own traumatic war-time experiences, was unable even on her death bed to share her experiences. Nevertheless she was able to establish, eventually, an emotionally rich relationship with her son Martin.

We still see how institutions and individuals deny any knowledge of abuse, whether in the family, in institutions, in homes, in churches. Even though Alice Miller was far from being a good mother to her children, while they were growing up, she still contributed very much to our present knowledge of the traumatic after-effects of child abuse on the grown-up victim of the abuse.

"day-glo"

19 THE GLOWING SPIRIT

Spirituality and the 21st Century.

"This is the dawning of the age of Aquarius..." London in the 1960s was really glowing with 'day-glo' paints, with the multi-coloured fashion on Carnaby Street, with the hippies, it did often look as if there was a new age dawning. Open-air concerts were full of people enjoying themselves, glowing with happiness. Fantasy or reality? Really a bit of both. Lots of things were new, society was really in a state of flux, Britain was no longer the centre of an empire but was beginning to think about developing trade and even cultural relationships with Europe, that is with continental Europe. For the very first time there was an inkling of a possibility of an eye-level meeting with other cultures! Even though the United States of America, France and Germany had outbreaks of violence when confronted with alternative lifestyles, Britain was remarkably peaceful – even the Police were very friendly and cooperative when dealing with, for example, the huge increase in people and traffic around Glastonbury during the early festivals.

For the first time, or so it seemed, since the second World War, Britain was glowing with life, love and hope for many. By all accounts, Britain and particularly London got caught up in a similar state during the celebrations around the Olympic Games in 2012.

Spiritism or as it's sometimes called, spiritualism, was a movement that caught the imagination and interest of the Victorians. Sir Arthur Conan Doyle was one of the leading proponents in Britain, whereas Madame Blavatsky and Rudolf Steiner were responsible for propagating various offshoots, such as the Theosophical Society and, in continental Europe, the Anthroposophy movement.

Steiner founded the Waldorf School movement, which is still very influential in Germany.

Apart from various theories about spirits of dead persons trying to communicate with the living, one interesting idea was that of an energetic envelope surrounding the physical body which, under particular circumstances, manifested itself as a glowing phenomenon around the person.

This is a theme that has kept recurring in various forms for thousands of years, from halos around ancient Egyptian painted figures, to halos around heads of Christian saints, up to Wilhelm Reich, an Austrian psychoanalyst who was excluded from the international psychoanalytic scene, mainly because of his theories about an energy body extending outside the physical body. Reich died in the 1960s in the USA but some of his ideas still influence theories in the realm of psychosomatic psychotherapy.

Invisible energy fields is a theme that stretches from China in the East, with Acupuncture being a manifestation within the human body and Feng Shui focussing on environmental energy patterns and their influence, both positive and negative, on individual human beings as well as human communities, and to Ley Lines in the West. Ley lines and their patterns are part of various 'pseudo-scientific' or metaphysical theories concerning the geometric patterns underlying the geographical positions of various sites that have been deemed to be of particular significance over the centuries in relation to religious or spiritual ceremonies.

Even though the author John Michell developed Alfred Watkins' concept of ley lines and sought a connection to Fey Shui, the various theories around ley lines have received little interest or recognition from the scientific community, leading to them being labelled 'pseudo scientific'. This is in contrast to Acupuncture which has slowly been accepted in orthodox medical circles and is, certainly in Germany, a recognised medical treatment.

I first visited Barcelona in 1970 and was not very impressed by what I saw in those pre-Olympic Games days. 2013 brought me back to the city and I was blown away by its attractiveness, but what impressed me most of all was a visit to Gaudi's masterpiece, the Sagrada Familia Cathedral. In the very highest corner of this amazing basilica church was a glowing triangle of diaphanous light of a golden yellow hue. For me, and from what I have read, that was Gaudi's intention; it truly represented that indefinable something that is variously called God, Allah, the Creative Spirit, that mysterious Soul that seems to be a common factor in all human beings.

Glow has been used for thousands of years to try to symbolise holiness or wholeness. We see it in the ancient Egyptian pictures of the rising sun as being the creative energy behind all life, with its constant recurring cycle of life and death every morning and evening.

We see it in the filigree light openings in the walls of the

Taj Mahal.

We see it in various poetic references to a "secret glow of light" in the heart of human beings.

We even see it in references to the football star David Beckham with 'Golden Balls' being capable of creating images not only of wealth and sexual prowess but also of a god-hero like quality!

The holy grail as a source of holy glow. Amongst the various stories circulating around the holy grail there is at least one theory that links the holy grail to a woman, to Mary, the virgin mother of Jesus Christ. Now it does not take a great deal of imagination to associate a woman with a vessel of some kind, prime examples are the amphora of ancient Greece and Rome. The next stage would be to label the vessel holy. As it is holy it would be natural to expect it to glow! Next time you are in Glastonbury, look up Chalice Well and its association with the Holy Grail. One can look at the holy grail as glowing, because it once held the blood, the holy blood of Jesus Christ and also because it represents the primary vessel from whom came Jesus Christ, and that is Mary, the holy mother.

Just as the Virgin Mary is the most important woman ever for the Roman Catholic Church, there are various women in other cultures who are famous, because of the sons they bore. One example is the goddess Isis, the mother of Horus, the patron god of the ancient Egyptians, sometimes looked at as the original Pharao. Then there is the matter of Olympia, the mother of Alexander the Great who, so the story goes, was impregnated by the gods on the eve of her marriage to Philip. According to another story, the mother of Constantine, the first Christian emperor and one of the chief architects of the Roman Catholic church, was Saint Helena, daughter of one of the ancient kings of

Britain, King Cole. He was later immortalised in the nursery rhyme 'Merry King Cole'.

Muslim architecture has traditionally used building techniques to transform harsh sunlight into mellow glows of light. During the course of researching for this book I came across a fellow Welshman who was also interested in glowing light within the Muslim architecture tradition. He was Owen Jones, a 19th century architect who co-designed the Crystal Palace, originally erected in Hyde Park, London to house the Great Exhibition of 1851, but who made his name and reputation as an expert in Arab and Moorish architecture and the author of the seminal design sourcebook, The Grammar of Ornament, published in 1856.

Our inner life is important even whilst asleep and dreams are a possible source of information about our not so conscious wishes and needs as well as anxieties or worries. Try looking closely at any dreams that refer to light or glowing.

Many pictorial representations of Buddha show his head glowing, sometimes with flames from a fire behind him. It's interesting that glow and glowing in various forms keeps on manifesting itself throughout history in various religious contexts. C. G. Jung's concepts of archetype and the collective unconscious fit in well with the universal and global character of glow and glowing.

Many people associate Quakers with porridge oats, puritanical beliefs or even with using horses and carts rather than cars. None are true, incidentally! However, one central aspect of Quaker belief is that of a common glow of inner light in every human body, whatever their skin, race or cultural affinities. This is the glowing spirit that has powered various Quaker social reform movements, notably in the fields of after-war care, mental health and prison reform.

The glowing spirit seems to play an important role in the lives of those persons who take their spiritual life seriously, whether within or without any organised religious framework.

The whole concept of glow seems to me to represent the interface of mind, body and soul, based on the ancient idea that if they are in harmony with each other then all is in order. Which leads to the conclusion that, if the time and place are also appropriate, we are on the way towards glowing!

*to
mor
row*

20 WHAT NEXT?

Who knows except you.

First thing in the morning, look into the mirror. Do you like what you see? Would you really enjoy spending the rest of the day with this person? Look at the eyes. Do they glow? Would you like to spend the rest of your life with this person? If not, why not?

What do like about Monday mornings? What! Yes, you heard, what do you like about Mondays? Nothing? Well, please change that attitude because Monday mornings are the most important mornings ever. Yes indeed. If you have a good sleep Sunday night, wake up full of energy on Monday, get up 30 minutes earlier than normal, do your pre-breakfast work out, whether running, yoga or whatever, then enjoy your breakfast you will be amazed, yes amazed how good your week will be. Don't believe it? You don't have to believe, you just have to try it out and experience how you feel, then and only then, can you determine whether you will be amazed.

What is right for you? What is the right food for you?
Some years ago an American Naturopath Peter d'Adamo
wrote a fascinating book about using blood groups as a
nutrition guide. Its called 'Eat Right for your Type'. Have
a look at what he has to say, then try it out – you might be
pleasantly surprised at the results. Certainly, over the last
15 years or so, many people all over the world have found
it helpful as a guide to their own personal individual nutrition planning.

On a personal note, I was fascinated, after years of working hard to achieve my personal level of health, particularly through a raw food vegetarian plan, to discover that
my own particular blood group, according to d'Adamo's
theory, is particularly well suited to this regime. So, even
though it was not my starting point I feel good about suggesting you read "Eat right for your type" for some ideas
about building your own individual nutrition plan.

Is there such a thing as right thinking? In general, of
course, we are moving towards the realm of morals
and ethics, but if we restrict ourselves to the subject of
thinking and worrying we may well get some guidance
from current research in autism. One interesting aspect
of someone manifesting autistic symptoms is that they
behave as if they had no idea how the people around them
think, let alone feel. Most of us tend to spend quite a bit of
energy trying to figure out what others think about us, we
even worry about what others feel or what they might feel.
As far as worrying is concerned it's probably a good idea
to do an occasional 'reality check'. For example, if you find
yourself worrying that your friend X thinks badly of you
after you drank too much at her party, try just asking her.
If even the thought of asking her is too much for you, then
you really do have a problem. And really should consider
seeking psychotherapy with a competent practitioner.

Some people find themselves worrying about how to deal with someone who said something hurtful. One quite useful way to deal with this is to approach the other in a friendly and polite manner and say something along the lines of, "Excuse me, did you really mean to hurt me by what you said to me?". Now it might turn out that they really did, in which case you have a very concrete issue to address, but in many cases it will turn out that there was no intention at all to inflict pain on you.

Your pain was very real, but it was the product of your fantasy. It was your imagination that imbued the words of the other with the power to hurt you. That is why it is of utmost importance to check whether the other person is really interested in inflicting pain upon you, before starting to either worry or even before starting to plan how to hurt them back. Worry combined with imagination and fantasy, slowly simmering inside you, can lead to a very explosive process, leading in turn to a lot of unnecessary pain and suffering.

Usually if I do something or make something that's really good, I feel a nice glow inside me, sometimes approaching a feeling of pride or admiration for work done well. However, there have been times and instances where I was unable to express my admiration to my inner self and found myself getting upset with my environment, meaning people, community and friends. Upset because no one said anything. Upset because they seemed uninterested. Upset because they seemed to take it for granted that I would do it and do it well. But lo and behold, if anything went wrong, there would be lots of unhappy faces!

My first stage, before learning how to feed the inner glow was the following: Try saying to those around you, "I am so happy with this project. It turned out well. It did seem to be easy but there were some tricky moments where my experience in the field helped me a lot. So I feel quite pleased with myself at the moment."

And then be quiet.

Hope you enjoy the reaction.

Now, worry affects our bodies. Whether it causes harm to our bodies is another matter, a matter over which we have some control. This is an important question because it seems that a conscious approach to our own particular worry can indeed have a positive effect on our health.

For example, Jonathan had problems at work that he was not able to solve. At some point he had difficulty sleeping. After some weeks he suffered from a racing pulse, meaning that his heart rate was much too fast with no physical exertion. Jonathan visited his doctor. Later a specialist. The problem was that as soon as the various doctors started to care for him, the symptom disappeared! One day his doctor suggested psychotherapy and Jonathan came to see me. Maybe you can imagine what happened? Yes indeed, after some time we started to look at the work problems, which led to relationship conflicts and so on. After much hard therapeutic work on Jonathan's side he was able to sleep peacefully and his pulse returned to normal.

Well of course it is not only the body that is affected by worry, it also affects our thinking mind as well as our emotional feelings. During the course of this book we have looked at various ways to approach worry. Whatever else you do I can only recommend that you spend some of your energy on the following Formula:

M S N

MEDITATION: Meaning whatever you feel good with, from a very simple breathing exercise to Vipassana meditation. Basically it has to do with practising being here in the now, slowing down or even stopping thought processes, letting feelings and images come to the surface of your conscious mind... and simply looking at them, as opposed to reacting to them. Sounds simple but it isn't!

SPORT: Again we are looking at a wide range of activities from taking a walk to training for the next Olympic Games. Whatever you do to look after your own body helps to reduce the necessity of others having to do it for you, whether that's your local GP, the local hospital or your private insurance scheme. It is a very practical way of expressing self-responsibility.

NUTRITION: Means simply being aware of what you put into your mouth, hopefully with some knowledge of how it is going to affect your life, both in the short and long term.

Think about M S N!

Some people find it very useful to have a daily programme of tasks. If you are one of them, consider making M S N your daily task, whether you spend three minutes or three hours on your individual M S N programme.

Then there are others for whom its important to have a big goal in life. But big tasks are very often daunting. In fact the very thought of having or wanting to do something big and important can even make it very difficult to take that first step.

In that respect a daily 'to-do list' can be useful. There are various references, particularly in American popular literature from the late 19th Century and the first half of the 20th Century to a to-do list 'just for today'. This is the version published in the Boston Globe newspaper in 1921, authored by Frank Crane.

Here are ten resolutions to make when you awake in the morning.

They are Just for One Day. Think of them not as a life task but as a day's work.

These things will give you pleasure. Yet they require will power. You don't need resolutions to do what is easy.

1. Just for Today, I will try to live through this day only, and not tackle my whole life-problem at once. I can do some things for twelve hours that would appal me if I felt I had to keep them up for a lifetime.

2. Just for Today, I will be Happy. This assumes that what Abraham Lincoln said is true, that "most folks are about as happy as they make up their minds to be". Happiness is from within; it is not a matter of Externals.

3. Just for Today, I will Adjust myself to what Is, and not try to Adjust everything to my own desires. I will take my

family, my business, and my luck as they come, and fit myself to them.

4. Just for Today, I will take care of my Body. I will exercise it, care for it, and nourish it, and not abuse it nor neglect it; so that it will be a perfect machine for my will.

5. Just for Today, I will try to strengthen my mind, I will study. I will learn something useful, I will not be a mental loafer all day. I will read something that requires effort, though and concentration.

6. Just for Today, I will exercise my Soul. In three ways, to wit:

(a) I will do somebody a good turn and not get found out. If anybody knows of it, it will not count.

(b) I will do at least two things I don't want to do, as William James suggests, just for exercise.

(c) I will not show any one that my feelings are hurt. They may be hurt, but Today I will not show it.

7. Just for Today, I will be agreeable. I will look as well as I can, dress as becomingly as possible, talk low, act courteously, be liberal with flattery, criticize not one bit nor find fault with anything, and not try to regulate nor improve anybody.

8. Just for Today, I will have a Programme. I will write down just what I expect to do every hour. I may not follow it exactly, but I'll have it. It will save me from the two pests Hurry and Indecision.

9. Just for Today, I will have a quiet half hour, all by myself, and relax. During this half hour, some time, I will think of God, so as to get a little more perspective to my life.

10. Just for Today, I will be Unafraid. Especially I will not be afraid to be Happy, to enjoy what is Beautiful, to love and to believe that those I love love me.

Some of you are maybe thinking that science is developing so quickly that it will not be long before we can switch off our worries and turn on our glow at will. Think again! Neuroscience gets lot of media attention but it does seem important to constantly remind ourselves that we are somewhat more than our brain and its functions.

So, what is the big secret? Could it be love?

Well, don't forget that love can be something other than the romantic love of the old Hollywood films!

In various religions and philosophies, there is the concept of 'loving kindness', referring to a practical way of living, which takes a benevolent and charitable attitude towards other human beings or even, indeed any living being.

PS: Don't believe everything you read, doubt even the things that seem believable to you. Check your emotional experiences, believe what you can and constantly doubt the truth of what you believe.

In this day and age it seems pretty superfluous to have an index when you can so easily do your own up to date research on google or any other search engine like duckduckgo.com.

If you really get stuck you could contact the author through www.snowdragon.pw

About the author

Bryn Jones was born in Caernarfon, Wales in 1938. He
was educated at Sir Hugh Owen School and attended
Liverpool College of Technology, London University,
Naturopathy Training Centre and C.G.Jung Institute
in Zurich. After a spell working as a design engineer in
the UK, he changed course, re-studied and later spent
more than a quarter century as a naturopath and analytic
psychotherapist in Germany.
Though he divides his time between Wales and
continental Europe, he feels most at home in Wales where
he now does most of his writing.

9 781721 969678